GRAVES' DISEASE
DIET COOKBOOK
FOR BEGINNERS

Essential Recipes for Managing Symptoms and Improving Thyroid Health Through Nutritional Balance

Kingsley Klopp

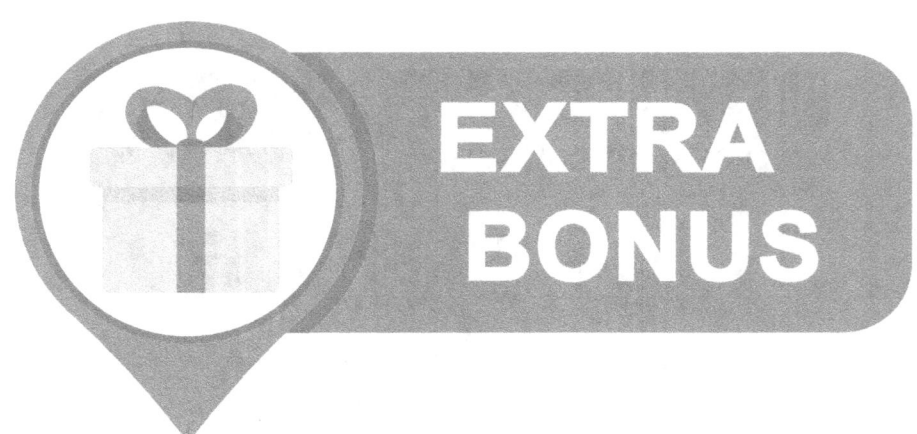

1. Weekly Meal Planner Journal
2. E-book with full color pictures

COPYRIGHT 2024
KINGSLEY KLOPP
ALL RIGHTS
RESERVED

Table of Contents

Introduction..7

Understanding Your Condition
- What is Graves' Disease?..9
- How Diet Can Help Manage Graves' Disease.................................10
- Symptoms of Graves' Disease..11
- How Graves' Disease Affects the Body.......................................12
- The Role of the Thyroid in Your Health....................................14

Dietary Principles for Graves' Disease
- Nutrients Important for Thyroid Health...................................16
- Foods to Include..18
- Foods to Avoid..20

Breakfast Recipes
Quinoa Porridge..22
Gluten-Free Oatmeal..23
Buckwheat Pancakes..24
Smoothie Bowl...25
Chia Pudding...26
Baked Sweet Potato...27
Avocado Toast...28
Muffins..29
Turkey Bacon Wraps..30
Greek Yogurt Parfait...31
Savory Oatmeal..32
Rice Cakes...33
Almond Flour Crepes...34
Pumpkin Porridge...35
Zucchini Bread..36
Coconut Yogurt..37
Mushroom and Spinach Frittata..38
Kale and Sweet Potato Hash..39
Apple Cinnamon Millet Bowl..40
Sautéed Greens..41
Polenta...42
Carrot Cake Oatmeal...43

Poultry Recipes

Grilled Chicken Salad..44
Turkey Meatballs..45
Chicken Stir-Fry..46
Roasted Turkey Breast..47
Chicken Soup..48
Baked Chicken with Herbs...49
Chicken Curry...50
Poached Chicken Breast...51
Turkey Stuffed Bell Peppers...52
Baked Turkey Meatloaf...53
Chicken Vegetable Kebabs...54
Stuffed Turkey Breast...55
Chicken Paillard..56
Turkey Skillet..57
Chicken Piccata..58
Roast Chicken with Thyme..59
Turkey Soup..60
Chicken Caesar Salad...61
Slow Cooker Turkey Breast..62
Turkey and Vegetable Stew..63
Grilled Chicken Caesar Wrap...64
Lemon Garlic Turkey Cutlets...65

Vegetables

Roasted Carrot and Ginger Soup...66
Sautéed Garlic Green Beans...67
Spiced Roasted Butternut Squash..68
Grilled Asparagus with Lemon...69
Zucchini Noodles with Pesto...70
Kale Salad with Avocado and Almonds.....................................71
Spinach and Mushroom Quiche...72
Beet and Carrot Slaw..73
Grilled Eggplant with Herbs..74
Vegetable Kabobs on the Grill...75
Spicy Stir-Fried Cabbage..76
Watercress and Pear Salad..77
Balsamic Roasted Beetroot...78
Swiss Chard and Lentil Stew..79
Herbed Potato Salad...80

Asian Cucumber Salad..81
Sautéed Rainbow Chard with Garlic...82
Grilled Zucchini Rolls with Herbed Cheese..83

Beef & Pork Recipes
Beef Stir-Fry...84
Pork Tenderloin...85
Beef and Vegetable Soup..86
Beef Stroganoff...87
Pork Chops with Apples and Onions..88
Italian Meatballs...89
Beef Kabobs..90
Pork and Sweet Potato Stew...91
Pork Loin Roast...92
Balsamic Glazed Beef..93
Spiced Pork Ribs...94
Beef Bourguignon..95
Pork Scallopini..96
Beef Chili...97
Ginger Pork Stir-Fry...98
Beef Brisket...99
Pork Carnitas..100
Beef Tenderloin with Herb Crust...101
Pork Vegetable Soup...102
Beef Goulash...103
Beef Ragout..104
Herb-Crusted Pork Medallions..105
Beef Fajitas...106

Fish & Seafood Recipes
Grilled Salmon with Lemon and Dill...107
Shrimp Stir-Fry with Mixed Vegetables..108
Baked Cod with Olive Tapenade..109
Pan-Seared Tuna Steaks...110
Seafood Paella with Brown Rice..111
Mussels in Tomato Garlic Broth...112
Crab Salad with Avocado and Cucumber..113
Halibut en Papillote...114
Scallops with Cauliflower Puree..115
Lemon Garlic Tilapia..116
Sardine Spread...117
Clam Chowder with Sweet Potatoes..118
Oyster Stew...119

Spicy Grilled Octopus..120
Salmon Burgers with Dill Yogurt Sauce..121
Prawn Curry with Coconut Milk...122
Smoked Haddock Omelette..123
Baked Sole with Herb Crust..124
Herring in Mustard Sauce...125

Meal Planner Journal..126

Dear Reader,

We understand that managing an autoimmune disorder is a deeply personal experience, which means the way your body responds to certain foods can be different from someone else's. That's why we encourage you to use these recipes as a starting point. Feel free to adjust ingredients and portions to better suit your specific health requirements and taste preferences. If you find yourself unsure about any changes or how a particular food might affect your condition, please consult with your healthcare provider. They can offer guidance tailored specifically to your health needs.

Furthermore, please note that the nutritional information provided with our recipes is approximate. Variations in specific ingredient types, brands, and preparation methods can all affect the final nutritional content of a dish. We strive to provide you with the most accurate information possible to help you make informed decisions about your diet, but a little personal tweaking may sometimes be necessary to align with your nutritional goals.

This cookbook isn't just about following recipes—it's about discovering what works best for your body, learning how to nourish yourself in a way that feels good, and hopefully, finding joy in the meals you prepare. So, take these recipes, tailor them as you see fit, and turn them into your own personal collection of Graves' disease-friendly favorites.

Additionally, if this cookbook has improved your cooking and dining experiences, we'd be delighted to hear about your adventures in an Amazon review. On the other hand, if you run into any problems with the recipes, please don't hesitate to contact us at **kloppkingsley@gmail.com**. We are committed to supporting you on your culinary journey.

Warm regards,

Kingsley Klopp

Introduction.

Welcome to the **"Graves' Disease Diet Cookbook for Beginners,"** a groundbreaking manual created to support you in overcoming the obstacles of using nutrition to manage Graves' disease. If you've recently been diagnosed with Graves' disease, or have been struggling with managing your symptoms, you know all too well how overwhelming and frustrating it can feel. This book is crafted to not only offer you comfort but also empower you with the knowledge and culinary tools to take control of your health.

Graves' disease, an autoimmune thyroid disorder, can turn your body into a battleground where excessive thyroid hormone production leads to a spectrum of symptoms that can disrupt daily life. From unexpected weight loss and nervousness to irritability and muscle weakness, the effects can be far-reaching and deeply distressing. But amidst these challenges lies a beacon of hope—your diet. *Why focus on diet, you might wonder?* Over the years, numerous studies and personal experiences have highlighted how specific dietary changes can significantly influence the progression and symptoms of autoimmune diseases, including Graves' disease. By embracing a diet tailored to reduce inflammation, minimize immune system triggers, and nourish your body, you can create a foundation for better health and improved quality of life. This cookbook is more than just a collection of recipes; it's a companion on your journey to wellness. We understand that changing your diet can be daunting, especially when facing a chronic condition. That's why we've designed this book to be a gentle, easy-to-follow introduction to eating for thyroid health. Each recipe has been carefully selected and crafted to ensure it is not only healthy but also delicious, simple to make, and satisfying. We believe that food should be enjoyed, not just consumed for health. From hearty breakfasts that set the tone for your day to nourishing dinners that satisfy and comfort after a long day, each dish is an opportunity to support your thyroid and overall health. We've included a variety of recipes to cater to different tastes and preferences, ensuring there's something for everyone. Whether you're a novice in the kitchen or looking to expand your cooking repertoire, these recipes will inspire confidence and creativity.

Moreover, this book doesn't just stop at recipes. We dive into the basics of Graves' disease, helping you understand the why behind each dietary recommendation.

You'll find practical tips on how to shop, cook, and eat out, making it easier to stick to your new diet without feeling restricted. We also understand the emotional toll of living with an autoimmune disease, so we offer strategies to cope with stress and maintain a positive outlook, essential components of any healing process.

Join us as we explore how simple changes in your kitchen can lead to significant changes in how you feel. Take the first step towards a healthier, more vibrant you. Embrace this new way of eating with open arms and an open heart, and let the "Graves' Disease Diet Cookbook for Beginners" guide you to a life where you are in control of your health, one delicious meal at a time.

Understanding Your Condition
What is Graves' Disease?

Graves' disease is an emotional rollercoaster for many who hear the diagnosis. It's an autoimmune disorder that primarily affects the thyroid, a small but mighty gland in the neck that influences almost every organ in your body. When you have Graves' disease, your immune system mistakenly attacks the thyroid, causing it to overproduce the hormones that regulate crucial bodily functions. This can feel like your body's own control center is in overdrive. Imagine your heart racing, hands trembling, and sleep fleeing despite intense fatigue—these are just a few symptoms that can profoundly disturb day-to-day life. It's not just a physical ordeal; the emotional and psychological toll can be just as challenging. Sufferers often experience anxiety and mood swings, adding an emotional dimension to the physical symptoms, making simple tasks seem daunting. The name **"Graves' Disease"** doesn't come from any grim origin but from Sir Robert Graves, the doctor who first described it in the early 19th century. While the name might sound a bit stark, the condition is manageable with the right medical care, including medications that regulate thyroid function, and in some cases, surgery or radioactive iodine treatments.

Beyond the medical facts, it's the human experience of Graves' disease that truly resonates. It's about the young mother striving for normalcy while grappling with palpitations, or the college student coping with unexpected weight loss and concentration troubles. It's about real people living their lives, facing each day with resilience, hoping for stability and a return to health.

How Diet Can Help Manage Graves' Disease.

Living with Graves' Disease can feel like being on an unending seesaw of physical and emotional highs and lows. Amidst this turmoil, diet emerges not just as a form of nourishment, but as a potential anchor, offering a semblance of control and empowerment. It's not a cure, but adjusting what you eat can significantly alleviate symptoms and improve quality of life, transforming food into a source of comfort and stability. Imagine this: Each meal is a chance to help soothe your overactive thyroid. Certain foods can dial down the intensity of your symptoms, while others might unknowingly crank it up. It's like having a toolkit where each tool is a different type of food that either soothes or provokes your condition. For someone grappling with Graves' Disease, understanding which foods to embrace and which to avoid can be a game-changer. Nutrient-rich foods that support immune system balance and thyroid health can be particularly beneficial. Selenium, found in Brazil nuts and seafood, and zinc, available in meat and dairy, are like tiny warriors supporting thyroid health. These aren't just nutrients; they're lifelines that help recalibrate your body's responses. Conversely, certain foods act almost like antagonists in this narrative. For instance, excessive iodine, which is pivotal for thyroid function, can paradoxically exacerbate Graves' symptoms when the thyroid is already overactive. Thus, moderating foods rich in iodine, like seaweed and shellfish, becomes a crucial strategy.

Moreover, diet isn't just about the physical. It plays a profound role emotionally. Sitting down to a meal tailored to manage your symptoms can bring a moment of peace, a feeling of normalcy when your body seems to be in constant rebellion. It's about crafting a daily routine that includes sipping on a calming herbal tea instead of a jitter-inducing coffee or enjoying a homemade, nutrient-packed smoothie that honors your body's needs. The journey with Graves' Disease is deeply personal, and integrating dietary changes is part of crafting a personalized path to well-being. This approach to diet is not just about avoiding and choosing foods; it's about embracing a lifestyle that brings holistic balance, nourishing both the body and the spirit. It's about reclaiming a sense of agency in your health narrative, one meal at a time.

Symptoms of Graves' Disease

Graves' disease, with its complex array of symptoms, can make those affected feel as if they are no longer in tune with their own bodies. This condition doesn't just disrupt physical health; it infiltrates every aspect of life, affecting emotional and psychological well-being with its unpredictable onslaught of symptoms. The most telltale symptom of Graves' disease is one that is often felt rather than seen: a *racing heart*. It's not just a flutter or a skip; it's like your heart is trying to break free from your chest, pounding relentlessly, disrupting calm and quiet moments. It can be frightening, a constant reminder that something inside isn't working as it should. Alongside this, there might be *trembling hands*, shaking not from cold or nerves, but from the ceaseless surge of thyroid hormones coursing through the veins. This tremor can turn simple tasks like holding a cup of coffee or writing a note into daunting challenges, stripping away layers of confidence and independence.

Weight loss is another common symptom, often rapid and unexplained. It can seem like a blessing at first, but the weight melts away not because of a healthy diet or exercise, but because your metabolism is in overdrive. Food is burned up at an alarming rate, and no amount of eating seems to fill the void. *Eyes* are the windows to the soul, but in Graves' disease, they narrate their own distressing story. Graves' ophthalmopathy can make the eyes bulge alarmingly, an uncomfortable and distressing symptom that doesn't just alter appearance but can also interfere with vision.

Sleep eludes many with this condition. Imagine lying in bed, exhausted yet unable to sleep, as your mind races along with your heart. Night after night, the lack of restorative sleep can wear down resilience, leaving you feeling perpetually tired yet wired, trapped in a frustrating cycle. *The skin*, too, tells its tale. It may become unusually smooth and thin, and even small amounts of heat can cause excessive sweating. It's as though the body's thermostat is broken, with every room feeling like a sauna.

Beyond the physical symptoms, Graves' disease can deeply impact emotional health. Anxiety and irritability can surge, often without warning, turning minor irritations into mountains of stress. This emotional volatility can strain relationships, adding a layer of social isolation to the physical challenges.

How Graves' Disease Affects the Body

Graves' disease, more than just a thyroid condition, sweeps through the body with a tidal wave of effects, touching nearly every system with its potent influence. The impact of this autoimmune disorder can be profound and pervasive, creating a symphony of changes that resonate through the physical, emotional, and mental realms of those it touches. At the heart of Graves' disease is the thyroid, a butterfly-shaped gland in the neck, small yet powerful in its role. When it's pushed into overactivity by the misguided assault of the immune system, it secretes an excess of thyroid hormones. These hormones are like the body's throttle, and when they flood the system, they push the body's metabolic rate into overdrive. This is not just a speeding up of functions but a relentless acceleration that can feel as if every part of you is running a marathon without a finish line. Imagine your heart, usually so steady and reliable, now beating rapidly and irregularly. This isn't just discomforting—it's exhausting and can be scary. It's like living with a drummer who constantly beats a fast rhythm, making calmness a memory and anxiety a constant companion. This heightened cardiac activity can lead to more serious heart conditions if not managed effectively, hanging over patients like a specter of potential heart disease.

The eyes are particularly vulnerable in Graves' disease. The same immune response that targets the thyroid can inflame and swell the tissues around the eyes. This isn't just a cosmetic issue; it's deeply affecting. It can make the eyes bulge, an appearance change that can cause distress and a profound emotional impact, altering how individuals see themselves and interact with the world. Vision can become a daily challenge, with dryness, irritation, and pressure that are both uncomfortable and unnerving. The skin and bones aren't spared either. The skin often becomes thin, fragile, and excessively sweaty, while the bones might start to lose their density more rapidly, a stealthy weakening that can lead to osteoporosis. These changes are insidious, creeping up silently and sometimes unnoticed until a sudden fracture or a look in the mirror brings the reality into sharp relief. Even the mind is ensnared by Graves' disease. The excess thyroid hormones can stir up anxiety and irritability, making emotional turbulence a regular feature of life. The mental fog, memory lapses, and concentration difficulties that often accompany Graves' disease can make sufferers feel alienated from their own thoughts, as if they're watching their mental acuity dissolve like mist.

Living with Graves' disease can feel like being caught in a storm with unpredictable winds and occasional clear skies. The pervasive impact of this condition can color every aspect of life, from the physical symptoms that are ever-present to the emotional and psychological challenges that weave through each day.

Understanding how Graves' disease affects the body is crucial not just for medical treatment but for empathy and support. It's a reminder that this condition is a multifaceted battle, not just with a physical illness but with the very essence of daily living. For those who navigate this storm, every small victory is a reclaiming of their own body and life's rhythm.

The Role of the Thyroid in Your Health

The thyroid gland, often unnoticed until it falters, plays a symphonic role in the concert of our body's functions. Nestled in the front of the neck, this butterfly-shaped gland is a master of metabolism, a conductor directing the energy that fuels our days and the systems that sustain our lives. Its influence stretches far and wide, affecting how we feel, think, and interact with the world around us. Understanding its role is not just about appreciating a biological function but about recognizing a cornerstone of our well-being. When the thyroid is in harmony with the rest of the body, its secretion of hormones—thyroxine (T4) and triiodothyronine (T3)—is a marvel of biological regulation. These hormones are the pace-setters, dictating how quickly or slowly our organs should work. They control the metabolic rate of almost every cell in the body, influencing how we burn calories, how our heart beats, and how we generate heat. It's like having a thermostat that ensures everything operates at just the right temperature. But the thyroid's influence doesn't end with metabolism. It reaches into the very core of our mental health. T3 and T4 hormones play critical roles in brain development and function, impacting our mood, memory, and cognitive abilities. When the thyroid is balanced, it can feel as though a fog has lifted from the mind, revealing a world in sharper focus and brighter colors. It supports our thoughts and emotions in a dance of neurological activity, helping to keep depression at bay and enabling us to handle stress more effectively.

The thyroid also casts its influence over our heart, driving the tempo at which it beats. It ensures that our heart muscles contract with the right force and frequency, managing blood flow and blood pressure. This isn't just a matter of numbers and medical metrics; it's about feeling vitality pulsing through our veins, about having the energy to pursue passions and embrace loved ones. For women, the thyroid weaves its effects into the very fabric of reproductive health. It regulates menstrual cycles and influences fertility. A woman with a well-balanced thyroid finds her body in a better rhythm, a harmony that can ease the journey through pregnancy and beyond. Yet, when the thyroid sings out of tune—whether overactive or underactive—the dissonance is felt deeply. Hypothyroidism can drape the body in weariness, weight gain, and chill, as if one is living in a world moving in slow motion, wrapped in an unshakeable cold.

Hyperthyroidism, on the other hand, is like a body in perpetual overdrive, a machine that can't stop even when exhausted, fueled by nervous energy and a heart that can't seem to slow down. The health of our thyroid is a linchpin in the delicate balance of our physical and emotional well-being. It's a testament to how intricately our bodies are designed, and how sensitive they are to the ebbs and flows of internal rhythms. To care for the thyroid is to care for the essence of our vitality, preserving the joy in our daily lives and the health in our future years.

Dietary Principles for Graves' Disease

Nutrients Important for Thyroid Health

When it comes to maintaining the delicate symphony of the body, the thyroid gland plays a pivotal role, and like any vital instrument, it requires the right nutrients to perform optimally. Ensuring your thyroid has the necessary nutrients is akin to nurturing the soul of your bodily functions—it impacts everything from your metabolic rate to your heart's rhythm and your emotional well-being.

The dance of thyroid health begins with **iodine**, a key player without which your thyroid cannot produce its essential hormones, T3 and T4. Imagine iodine as the foundational bricks of a building—without it, the structure of thyroid hormone production simply cannot stand. However, it's a delicate balance; too little leads to dysfunction, and too much can provoke the thyroid into an overactive state. It's about finding that sweet spot, much like tuning a guitar to achieve the perfect pitch.

Next in our nutrient ensemble is **selenium**, a powerful antioxidant that protects the thyroid gland from damage by free radicals, much like a faithful shield in battle. Selenium is crucial in converting T4 into T3, the more active hormone that your body can use. Picture selenium as a backstage technician in a play, ensuring that everything runs smoothly behind the curtains so that the performance can go on without a hitch.

Zinc plays its role with quiet importance, involved deeply in the synthesis of thyroid hormone. It's like the unsung hero behind the scenes, essential but often overlooked. Zinc ensures that the thyroid hormone gets where it needs to go and is converted into its active form, facilitating a myriad of bodily functions from cellular metabolism to new cell production.

Iron is another cornerstone for thyroid health, especially in how it supports the production of thyroid hormone. Lack of iron can be likened to a factory running low on raw materials; without it, the production line of thyroid hormones slows down, affecting everything from energy levels to temperature regulation.

Then there's **vitamin D**, often celebrated for its role in bone health but equally vital for the thyroid. Vitamin D helps regulate the immune system, which is particularly important in autoimmune conditions like Hashimoto's thyroiditis, where the body mistakenly attacks thyroid tissue. It acts much like a mediator, promoting peace and understanding in the complex immune system landscape.

Vitamin B12 is also indispensable, particularly for those with hypothyroidism, as deficiencies in B12 can mimic or exacerbate symptoms of low thyroid function. It contributes to nerve health and energy production, offering a boost like a cup of coffee in the morning—essential to kickstart your day.

Each of these nutrients plays a vital role in supporting thyroid health, contributing their unique strengths to ensure this gland can fulfill its critical functions. But it's not just about the biological roles they play; it's about the harmony they create, the sense of vitality they nurture. For those managing thyroid issues, focusing on these nutrients isn't just about following medical advice—it's about weaving a tapestry of health and well-being, thread by thread, meal by meal. It's a journey of nurturing not just a gland, but the very essence of life's quality.

Foods to Include

When managing thyroid health, particularly conditions like Graves' disease or Hashimoto's thyroiditis, the foods you choose to include in your diet are not just sustenance—they are tools for healing and harmony. Each meal can be a loving gesture towards your body, an offering of nutrients that support and soothe your thyroid, helping to restore balance and enhance well-being.

Seafood stands out in the culinary choir for its rich content of iodine and selenium. Imagine savoring a piece of baked salmon or a tender scallop—these aren't just delicious bites; they are laden with the iodine necessary for thyroid hormone production and the selenium that protects your gland from oxidative stress. It's like eating a melody that's both soothing and invigorating.

Nuts and seeds, especially Brazil nuts, sunflower seeds, and flaxseeds, are like little packets of nutritional gold. They offer selenium, which helps convert thyroid hormones to their active form, and healthy fats that support overall cell health. Integrating these into your diet can be as simple as sprinkling a handful on a morning bowl of yogurt or oatmeal, transforming an ordinary breakfast into a nourishing start to your day.

Dairy products also play a harmonious tune in this ensemble by providing both iodine and vitamin D. A glass of milk, a slice of cheese, or a spoonful of Greek yogurt can help maintain the calcium balance that might be disrupted by thyroid issues. It's comforting to know that such simple choices can bolster your health in profound ways.

Eggs are another versatile and valuable player. They contain iodine and selenium, and their protein helps keep you full and satisfied, stabilizing energy levels throughout the day. Whether boiled, poached, or scrambled, eggs bring a comforting presence to any meal, serving as a reminder that nourishment comes in simple, familiar forms.

Fruits and vegetables are vital, not just for their fiber and antioxidants but for their role in maintaining a healthy weight and reducing inflammation. Brightly colored vegetables and fruits like berries, carrots, and peppers aren't just a feast for the eyes; they're packed with nutrients that help fend off the oxidative stress that can accompany thyroid dysfunction.

Whole grains like oats, brown rice, and whole wheat provide fiber, which supports digestive health—a common concern for those with thyroid issues. They are the steady, comforting base in meals, helping to modulate blood sugar levels and sustain energy throughout the day.

Lean meats and poultry are excellent sources of zinc, which is crucial for thyroid function. Including chicken or turkey in your diet can be like adding a robust base note to the symphony of foods that support your thyroid, grounding your meals with substance and strength.

Incorporating these foods into your diet is like composing a daily symphony of flavors, colors, and textures that not only delight the palate but also bring peace and balance to your body. Eating well becomes a form of self-care, a way to cherish and support your body against the challenges of thyroid disease. Each meal is an opportunity to nourish not just the body but also the soul, reminding us that even in the midst of managing a health condition, there can be moments of joy and contentment at the dining table.

Foods to avoid

Navigating the world of food when managing a thyroid condition such as Graves' disease can sometimes feel like walking through a minefield. Each choice at the grocery store or meal at a restaurant carries weight, as some foods can exacerbate symptoms or interfere with thyroid function. Knowing which foods to avoid is not about restriction but about protection—shielding your body from substances that could disturb the delicate balance of your health.

Gluten often tops the list of foods to consider avoiding, especially for those with autoimmune thyroid diseases like Hashimoto's thyroiditis. For many, gluten can provoke inflammation or increase the risk of an autoimmune response. Imagine the body mistakenly identifying gluten as a threat, leading to increased inflammation that can spill over to affect the thyroid. Choosing gluten-free grains like quinoa or buckwheat can become an act of kindness toward your body, alleviating potential distress and promoting digestive peace.

Soy products can also be contentious. While soy is celebrated in many health circles for its benefits, it contains goitrogens—substances that can interfere with thyroid hormone production by inhibiting the body's iodine absorption. Foods like tofu, soy milk, and edamame might need to be limited, especially if consumed raw. Think of it as sidestepping a food that could throw a wrench in the finely tuned machinery of your thyroid function.

Cruciferous vegetables such as broccoli, cauliflower, and kale, though packed with nutrients, also contain goitrogens. Cooking these vegetables can neutralize much of their goitrogenic activity, transforming them from potential disruptors to beneficial allies in your diet. It's like gently coaxing a song from a difficult instrument, making it harmonize with your body's needs rather than work against them.

Excessive iodine can be a double-edged sword for thyroid health. While adequate iodine is crucial, too much can exacerbate hyperthyroidism or Graves' disease. High-iodine foods like kelp or other seaweeds should be consumed cautiously. It's about finding balance, like adjusting the volume of a speaker that's set too loud; you want enough sound to fill the room, not overwhelm it.

Caffeine and alcohol can aggravate symptoms of thyroid disorders by increasing anxiety, disrupting sleep, and affecting the absorption of thyroid medication. Reducing or avoiding caffeine and alcohol can feel like smoothing out the edges of a day filled with spikes of energy and dips of exhaustion, leading to a more even, calm experience.

Sugars and highly processed foods should be minimized as they can contribute to weight gain and instability in blood sugar levels, complicating the management of thyroid disorders. These foods are like the high and lows of a tumultuous relationship—thrilling in the moment but ultimately disruptive and draining.

Choosing to avoid these foods is a profound act of self-care, a decision to prioritize your long-term health over momentary pleasures. It's about nurturing your body, understanding its vulnerabilities, and creating an environment where it can thrive despite the challenges posed by thyroid disease. Each meal becomes a testament to resilience, a deliberate choice to support your well-being, and embrace a lifestyle that fosters stability and health.

Breakfast Recipes

1. Quinoa Porridge
Ingredients:
- 1 cup quinoa, rinsed
- 2 cups water
- 1 cup unsweetened almond milk
- 1 apple, peeled and diced
- 1/2 teaspoon cinnamon
- 2 tablespoons honey or maple syrup
- 1/4 cup chopped nuts (such as almonds or walnuts)
- 1/4 cup fresh berries

Instructions:
1. Combine quinoa and water in a medium saucepan. Bring to a boil, then reduce heat to low and simmer covered until the water is absorbed (about 15 minutes).
2. Stir in almond milk, diced apple, and cinnamon. Simmer for an additional 5 minutes or until the porridge is creamy and apples are tender.
3. Serve warm, topped with honey or maple syrup, nuts, and fresh berries.

Nutrition Info (per serving, serves 4):
- Calories: 280
- Protein: 8 g
- Carbohydrates: 50 g
- Fat: 7 g
- Fiber: 6 g

Cooking Time: 20 minutes

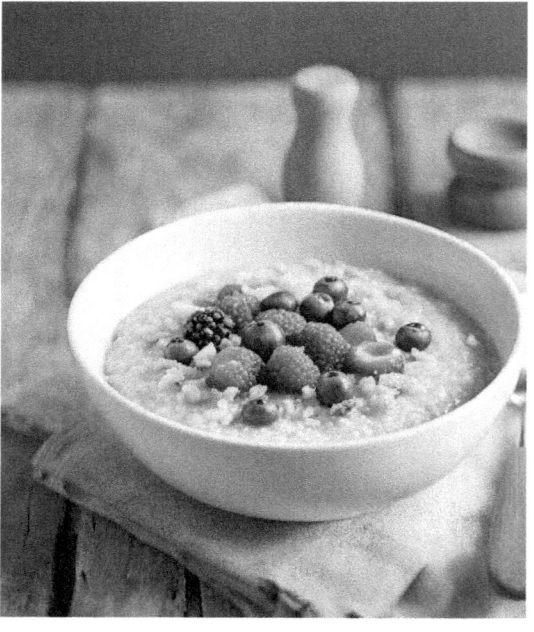

2. Gluten-Free Oatmeal

Ingredients:
- 1 cup gluten-free oats
- 2 cups water or dairy-free milk
- 1 banana, sliced
- 1 tablespoon chia seeds
- 1/2 teaspoon vanilla extract
- 1/4 cup raisins
- 1 tablespoon honey or maple syrup

Instructions:
1. Bring the water or milk to a boil in a saucepan. Add oats and reduce heat.
2. Simmer for 10 minutes, stirring occasionally, until the oats are soft.
3. Stir in banana, chia seeds, vanilla, and raisins. Cook for another 5 minutes.
4. Serve warm, drizzled with honey or maple syrup.

Nutrition Info (per serving, serves 2):
- Calories: 340
- Protein: 7 g
- Carbohydrates: 67 g
- Fat: 5 g
- Fiber: 9 g

Cooking Time: 15 minutes

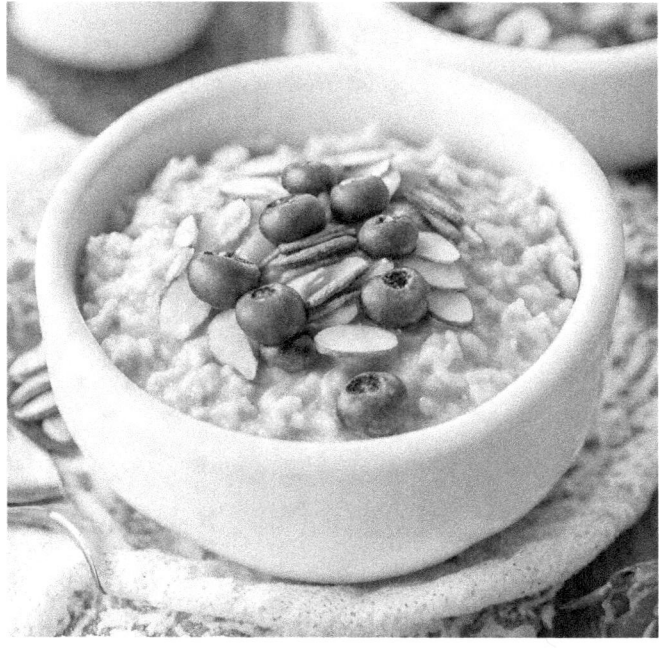

3. Buckwheat Pancakes

Ingredients:
- 1 cup buckwheat flour
- 1 teaspoon baking powder
- 1/2 teaspoon cinnamon
- 1 tablespoon honey or maple syrup
- 1 egg
- 1 cup almond milk
- 1 teaspoon vanilla extract
- 1/2 cup blueberries

Instructions:
1. In a bowl, mix buckwheat flour, baking powder, and cinnamon.
2. In another bowl, whisk together honey, egg, almond milk, and vanilla.
3. Combine the wet and dry ingredients, stirring until smooth.
4. Fold in blueberries.
5. Heat a non-stick pan over medium heat and pour 1/4 cup batter for each pancake.
6. Cook until bubbles form on the surface, then flip and cook until golden brown.

Nutrition Info (per serving, serves 4):
- Calories: 190
- Protein: 6 g
- Carbohydrates: 34 g
- Fat: 3 g
- Fiber: 5 g

Cooking Time: 20 minutes

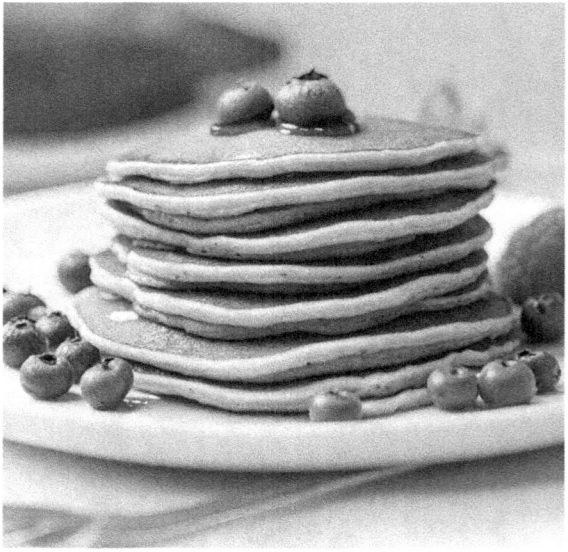

4. Smoothie Bowl

Ingredients:
- 1 frozen banana
- 1/2 cup frozen berries
- 1 cup spinach leaves
- 1 tablespoon flaxseed meal
- 1/2 cup coconut water
- 1/4 cup granola (gluten-free)
- 1 tablespoon pumpkin seeds
- 1 tablespoon coconut flakes

Instructions:
1. Blend the banana, berries, spinach, flaxseed meal, and coconut water until smooth.
2. Pour into a bowl and top with granola, pumpkin seeds, and coconut flakes.

Nutrition Info (per serving, serves 1):
- Calories: 350
- Protein: 8 g
- Carbohydrates: 60 g
- Fat: 10 g
- Fiber: 9 g

Cooking Time: 5 minutes

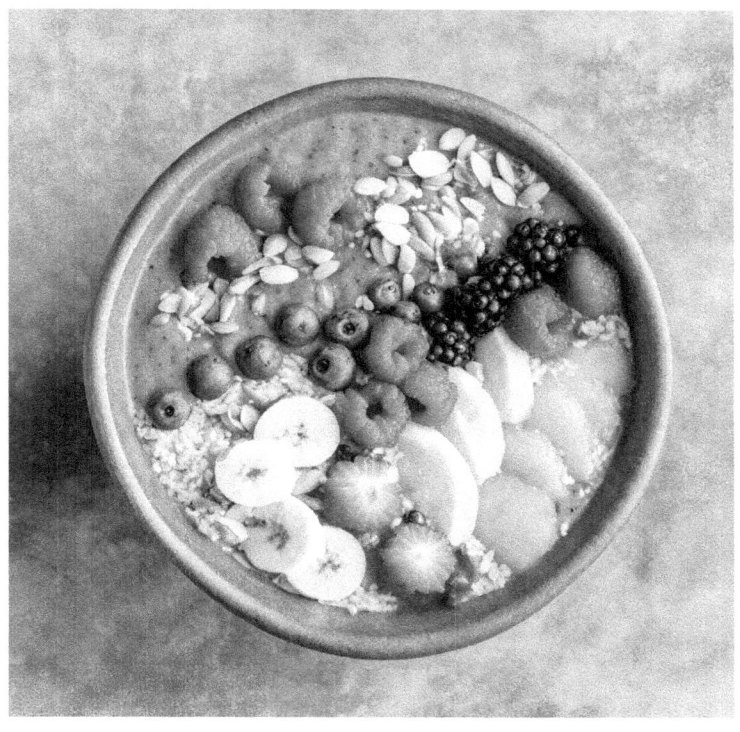

5. Chia Pudding

Ingredients:
- 1/4 cup chia seeds
- 1 cup unsweetened almond milk
- 1 tablespoon honey or maple syrup
- 1/2 teaspoon vanilla extract
- 1/2 cup mixed berries
- 1 tablespoon shredded coconut

Instructions:
1. In a bowl, mix chia seeds, almond milk, honey, and vanilla extract.
2. Stir well and let sit for 5 minutes, then stir again to prevent clumping.
3. Cover and refrigerate overnight.
4. Serve topped with mixed berries and shredded coconut.

Nutrition Info (per serving, serves 2):
- Calories: 220
- Protein: 5 g
- Carbohydrates: 28 g
- Fat: 11 g
- Fiber: 14 g

Cooking Time: Overnight (plus 10 minutes prep)

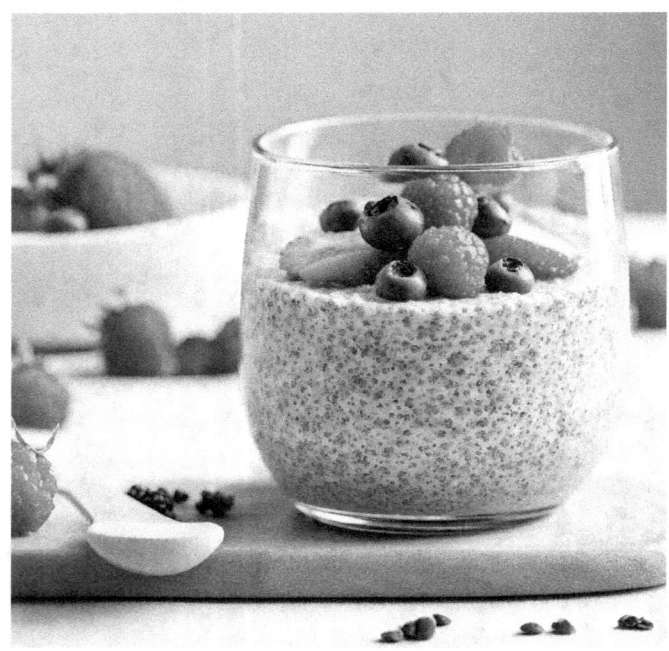

6. Baked Sweet Potato

Ingredients:
- 2 medium sweet potatoes, washed
- 1 tablespoon olive oil
- 1/2 teaspoon cinnamon
- 2 tablespoons almond butter

Instructions:
1. Preheat the oven to 400°F (200°C).
2. Prick the sweet potatoes with a fork and brush with olive oil.
3. Bake in the oven for 45-50 minutes until tender.
4. Split open and sprinkle with cinnamon, then top with almond butter.

Nutrition Info (per serving, serves 2):
- Calories: 290
- Protein: 5 g
- Carbohydrates: 45 g
- Fat: 11 g
- Fiber: 7 g

Cooking Time: 50 minutes

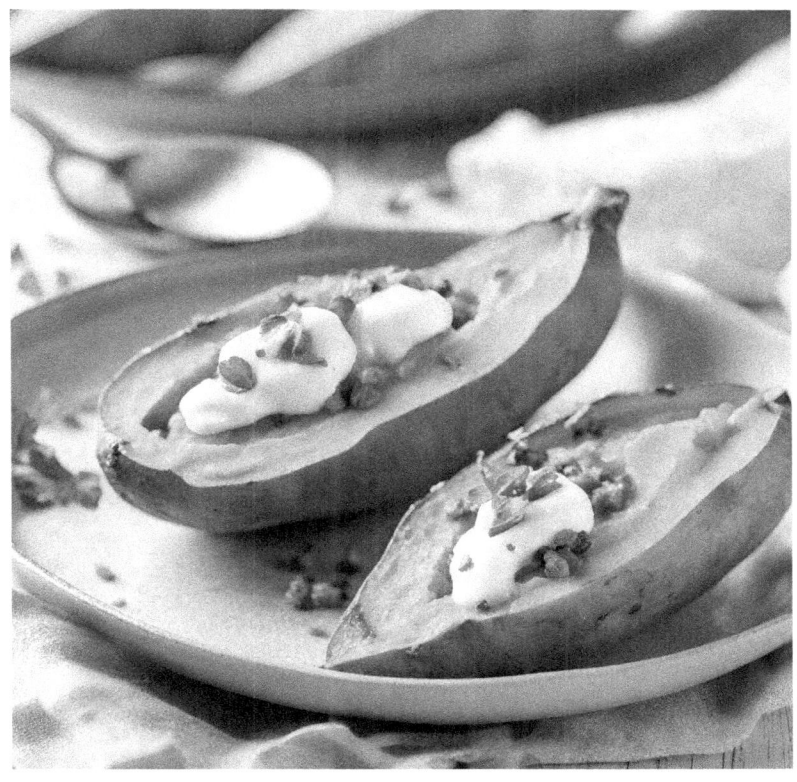

7. Avocado Toast

Ingredients:
- 2 slices of gluten-free bread
- 1 ripe avocado
- 1 tomato, sliced
- 1 teaspoon lemon juice
- Fresh herbs (such as basil or cilantro), chopped

Instructions:
1. Toast the gluten-free bread until golden and crispy.
2. Mash the avocado with lemon juice and spread on the toast.
3. Top with sliced tomato and sprinkle with fresh herbs.

Nutrition Info (per serving, serves 2):
- Calories: 250
- Protein: 5 g
- Carbohydrates: 27 g
- Fat: 15 g
- Fiber: 8 g

Cooking Time: 10 minutes

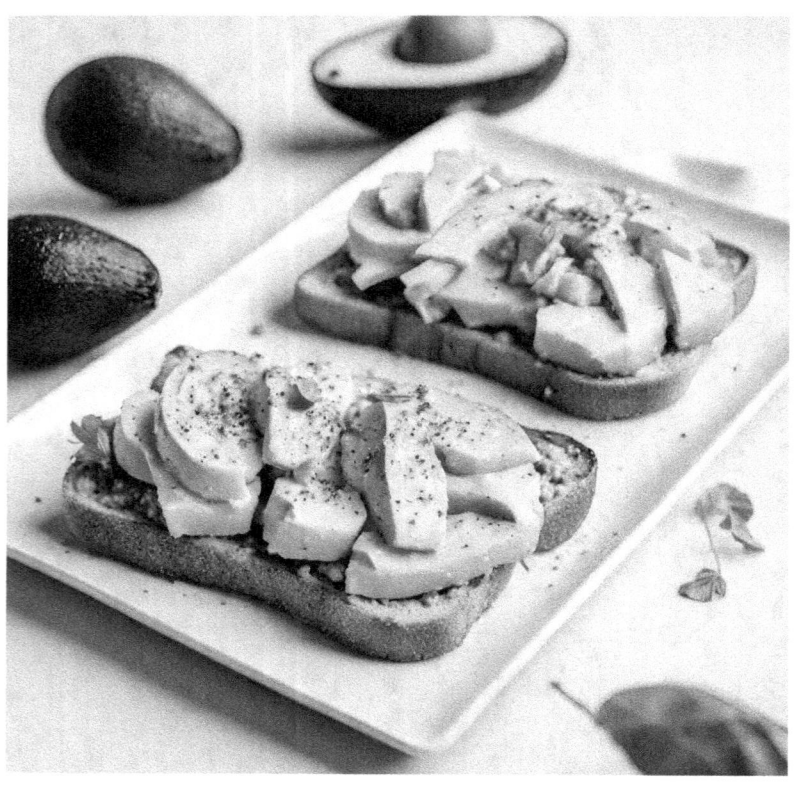

8. Egg Muffins

Ingredients:
- 6 eggs
- 1/2 cup chopped spinach
- 1/4 cup diced bell peppers
- 1/4 cup shredded carrots
- 1 tablespoon olive oil

Instructions:
1. Preheat the oven to 350°F (175°C).
2. Whisk eggs in a bowl with olive oil.
3. Stir in spinach, bell peppers, and carrots.
4. Pour into greased muffin tins and bake for 20-25 minutes until set.

Nutrition Info (per serving, serves 6):
- Calories: 100
- Protein: 7 g
- Carbohydrates: 2 g
- Fat: 7 g
- Fiber: 1 g

Cooking Time: 25 minutes

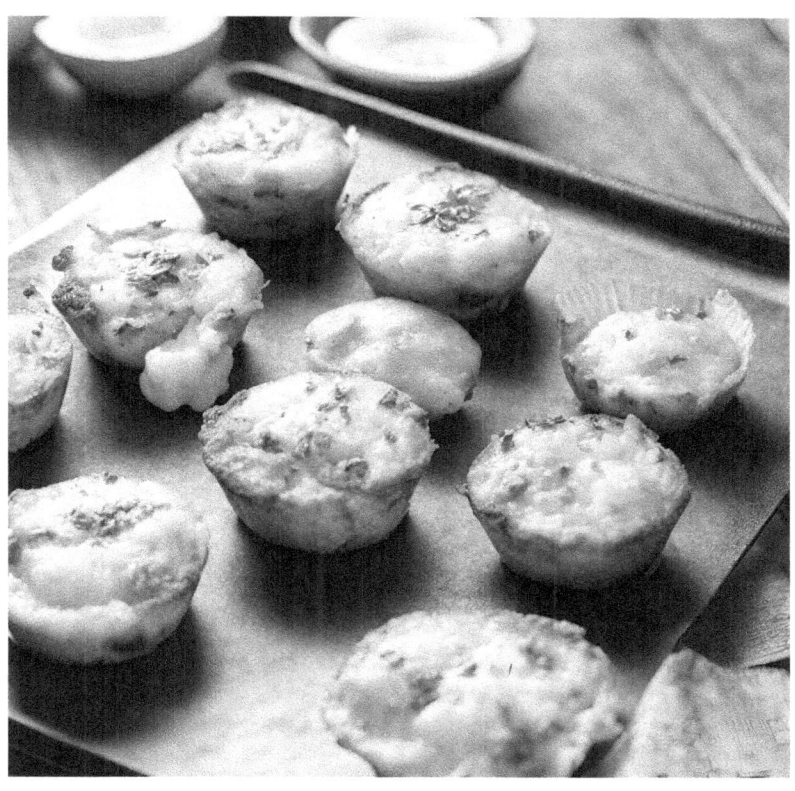

9. Turkey Bacon Wraps

Ingredients:
- 4 slices turkey bacon
- 4 lettuce leaves
- 1 tomato, sliced
- 1/4 cup sliced cucumber
- 1 tablespoon mustard

Instructions:
1. Cook turkey bacon until crisp.
2. Place each slice on a lettuce leaf, add tomato and cucumber slices.
3. Drizzle with mustard, wrap the lettuce around the fillings.

Nutrition Info (per serving, serves 4):
- Calories: 70
- Protein: 6 g
- Carbohydrates: 2 g
- Fat: 4 g
- Fiber: 1 g

Cooking Time: 10 minutes

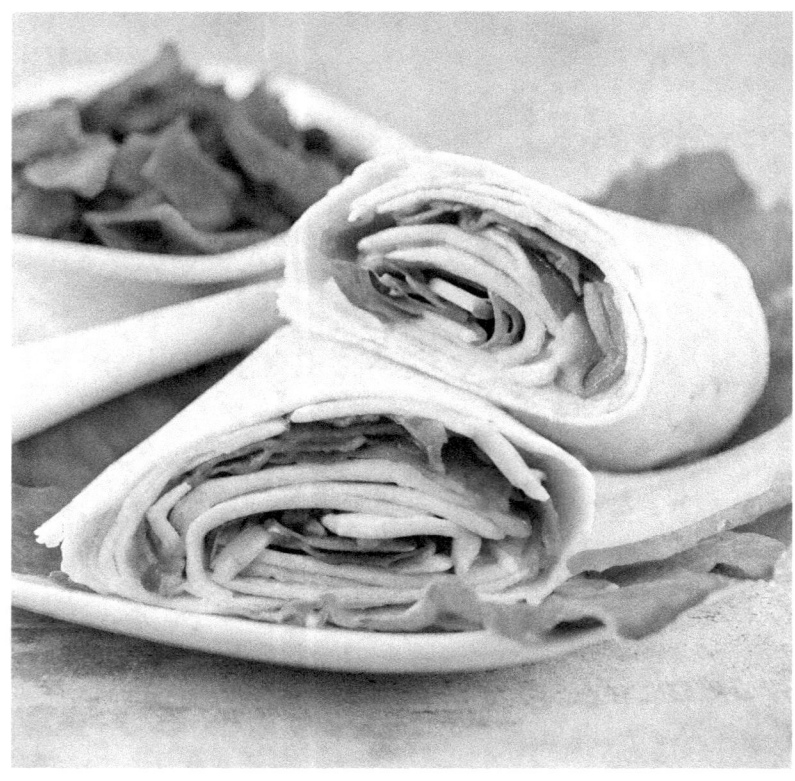

10. Greek Yogurt Parfait

Ingredients:
- 1 cup Greek yogurt, unsweetened
- 1/4 cup granola (gluten-free)
- 1/2 cup fresh berries
- 1 tablespoon honey or maple syrup

Instructions:
1. Layer Greek yogurt in a glass.
2. Top with granola, then berries.
3. Drizzle with honey or maple syrup.

Nutrition Info (per serving, serves 1):
- Calories: 320
- Protein: 25 g
- Carbohydrates: 36 g
- Fat: 10 g
- Fiber: 4 g

Cooking Time: 5 minutes

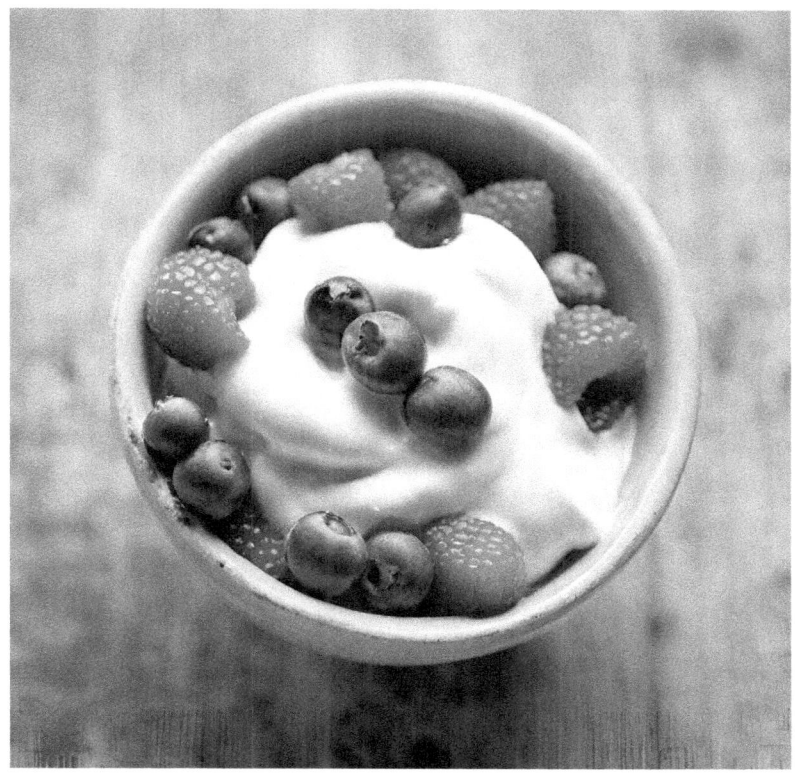

11. Savory Oatmeal

Ingredients:
- 1 cup steel-cut oats
- 3 cups water
- 1/2 cup chopped mushrooms
- 1/4 cup diced red bell pepper
- 1/4 cup grated zucchini
- 1 tablespoon olive oil
- Fresh herbs (such as thyme or parsley), chopped

Instructions:
1. Cook oats in water according to package directions until tender.
2. While the oats are cooking, sauté mushrooms, bell pepper, and zucchini in olive oil until soft.
3. Mix the sautéed vegetables into the cooked oatmeal.
4. Garnish with fresh herbs before serving.

Nutrition Info (per serving, serves 4):
- Calories: 150
- Protein: 5 g
- Carbohydrates: 23 g
- Fat: 5 g
- Fiber: 4 g

Cooking Time: 25 minutes

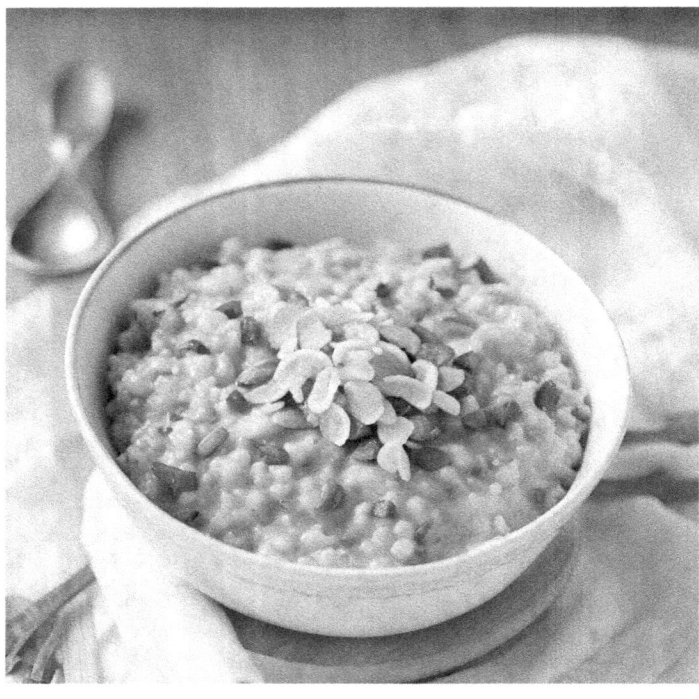

12. Rice Cakes

Ingredients:
- 4 plain rice cakes
- 2 tablespoons almond butter
- 1 banana, sliced
- 1/4 teaspoon cinnamon
- 1 tablespoon honey or maple syrup

Instructions:
1. Spread almond butter evenly on each rice cake.
2. Top with banana slices and sprinkle with cinnamon.
3. Drizzle with honey or maple syrup.

Nutrition Info (per serving, serves 4):
- Calories: 150
- Protein: 3 g
- Carbohydrates: 23 g
- Fat: 6 g
- Fiber: 2 g

Cooking Time: 5 minutes

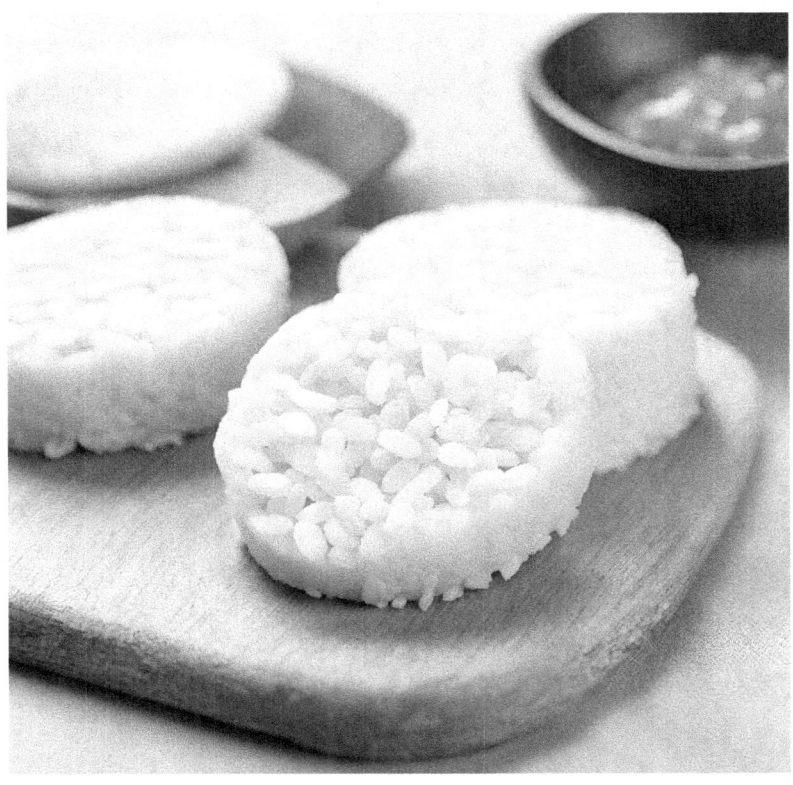

13. Almond Flour Crepes

Ingredients:
- 1 cup almond flour
- 2 eggs
- 1/2 cup almond milk
- 1 tablespoon honey or maple syrup
- 1/2 teaspoon vanilla extract
- Olive oil for cooking

Instructions:
1. Whisk together almond flour, eggs, almond milk, honey, and vanilla extract until smooth.
2. Heat a little olive oil in a non-stick pan over medium heat.
3. Pour a small amount of batter into the pan and swirl to spread evenly.
4. Cook for 1-2 minutes per side until golden brown. Repeat with remaining batter.

Nutrition Info (per serving, serves 4):
- Calories: 220
- Protein: 9 g
- Carbohydrates: 12 g
- Fat: 17 g
- Fiber: 3 g

Cooking Time: 20 minutes

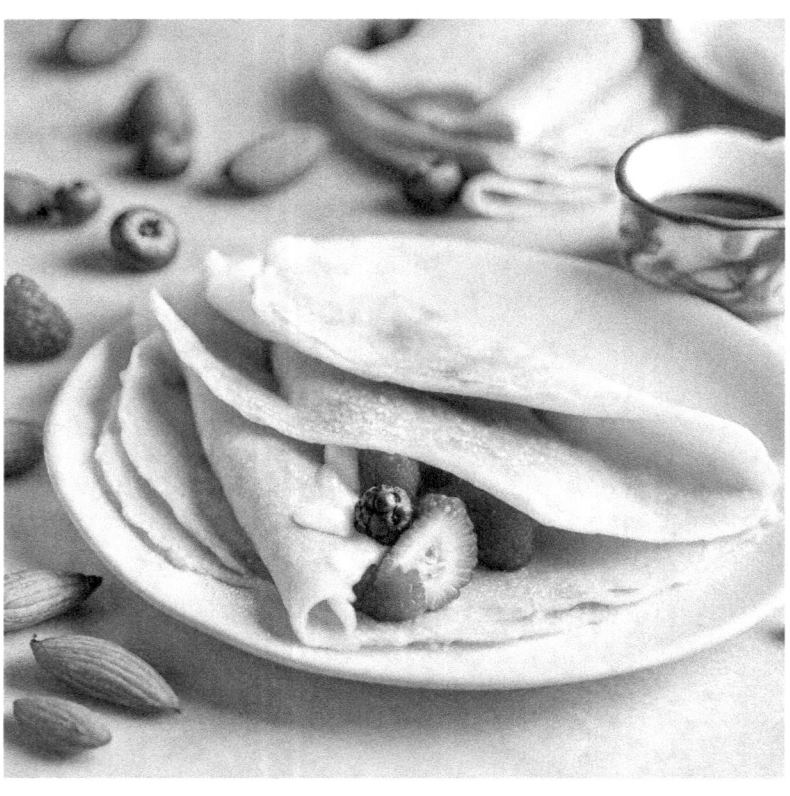

14. Pumpkin Porridge

Ingredients:
- 1 cup canned pumpkin puree
- 1 cup almond milk
- 1/2 teaspoon cinnamon
- 1/4 teaspoon nutmeg
- 1 tablespoon honey or maple syrup
- 1/4 cup chopped pecans

Instructions:
1. In a pot, combine pumpkin puree, almond milk, cinnamon, and nutmeg.
2. Cook over medium heat until heated through.
3. Serve hot, topped with honey and chopped pecans.

Nutrition Info (per serving, serves 2):
- Calories: 210
- Protein: 3 g
- Carbohydrates: 29 g
- Fat: 11 g
- Fiber: 7 g

Cooking Time: 10 minutes

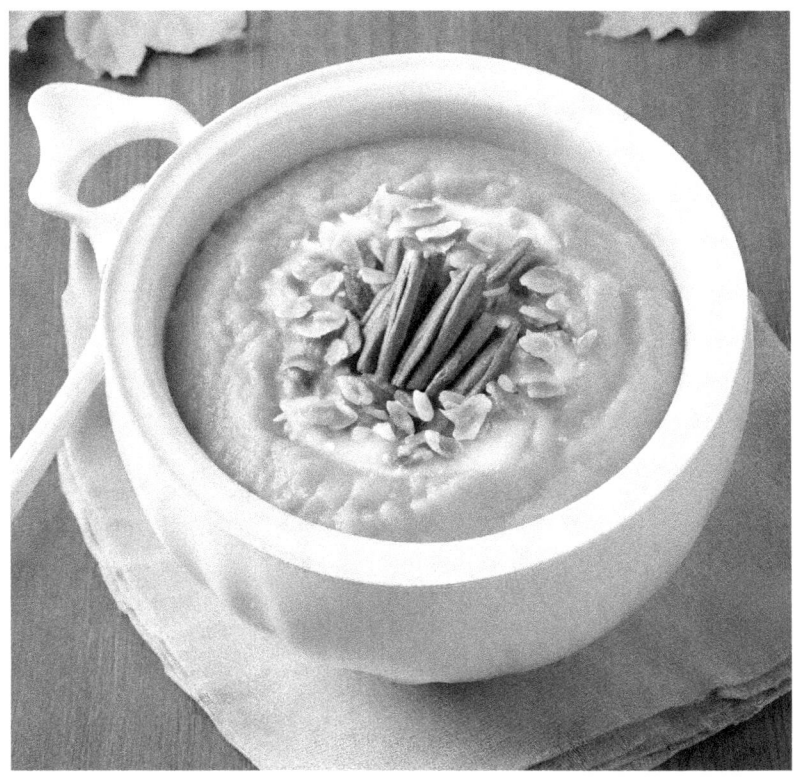

15. Zucchini Bread

Ingredients:
- 1 cup grated zucchini
- 1 cup almond flour
- 1/2 cup coconut flour
- 1/4 cup olive oil
- 1/4 cup honey or maple syrup
- 2 eggs
- 1 teaspoon baking soda
- 1 teaspoon cinnamon
- 1/2 teaspoon nutmeg

Instructions:
1. Preheat oven to 350°F (175°C).
2. Combine all ingredients in a bowl and mix until well blended.
3. Pour batter into a greased loaf pan.
4. Bake for 50 minutes or until a toothpick inserted into the center comes out clean.

Nutrition Info (per serving, serves 8):
- Calories: 210
- Protein: 6 g
- Carbohydrates: 20 g
- Fat: 13 g
- Fiber: 4 g

Cooking Time: 50 minutes

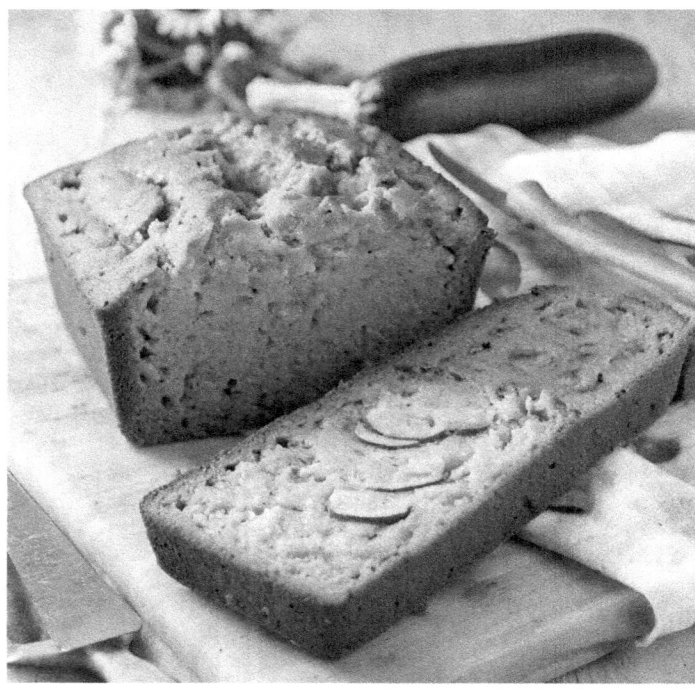

16. Coconut Yogurt

Ingredients:
- 2 cups of coconut milk
- 2 probiotic capsules
- 1 tablespoon maple syrup (optional, for sweetness)

Instructions:
1. Heat coconut milk to just warm to the touch, then whisk in the contents of probiotic capsules.
2. Transfer to a sterile jar and cover lightly with cheesecloth.
3. Let sit in a warm place for 24-48 hours, depending on how tangy you want your yogurt.
4. Once fermented, stir in maple syrup if using, and refrigerate to thicken.

Nutrition Info (per serving, serves 4):
- Calories: 120
- Protein: 1 g
- Carbohydrates: 3 g (without maple syrup)
- Fat: 12 g
- Fiber: 0 g

Cooking Time: 24-48 hours for fermentation

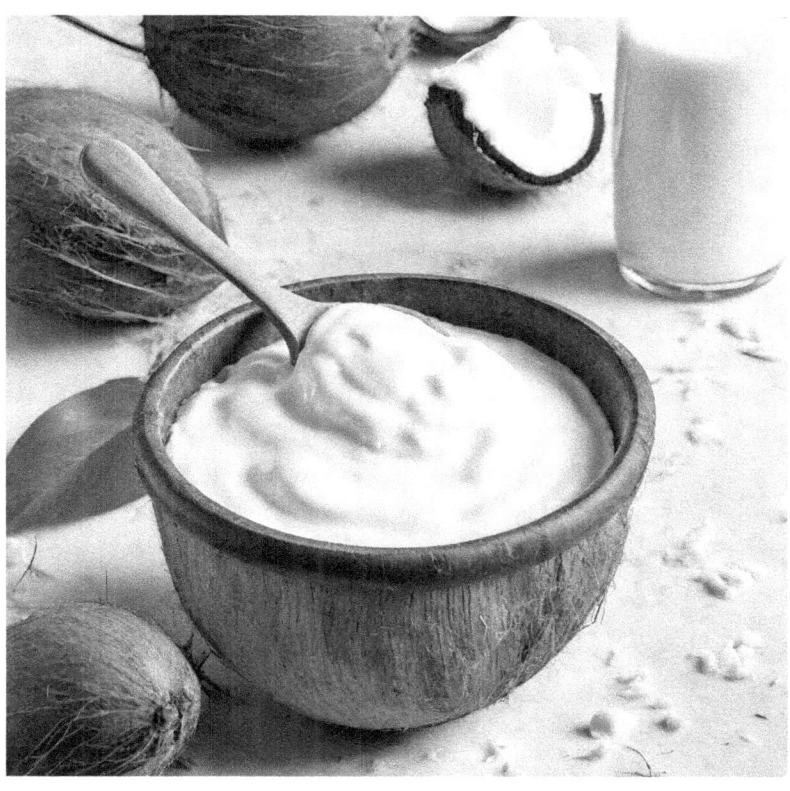

17. Mushroom and Spinach Frittata

Ingredients:
- 6 eggs
- 1 cup chopped mushrooms
- 1 cup fresh spinach
- 1/4 cup diced onions
- 2 tablespoons olive oil
- 1/4 cup almond milk

Instructions:
1. Preheat the oven to 375°F (190°C).
2. Sauté onions and mushrooms in olive oil until tender.
3. Add spinach and cook until wilted.
4. Whisk together eggs and almond milk, then pour over the vegetables in a skillet.
5. Cook for a few minutes without stirring, then transfer skillet to the oven.
6. Bake for 15-20 minutes or until the eggs are set.

Nutrition Info (per serving, serves 4):
- Calories: 180
- Protein: 11 g
- Carbohydrates: 4 g
- Fat: 14 g
- Fiber: 1 g

Cooking Time: 30 minutes

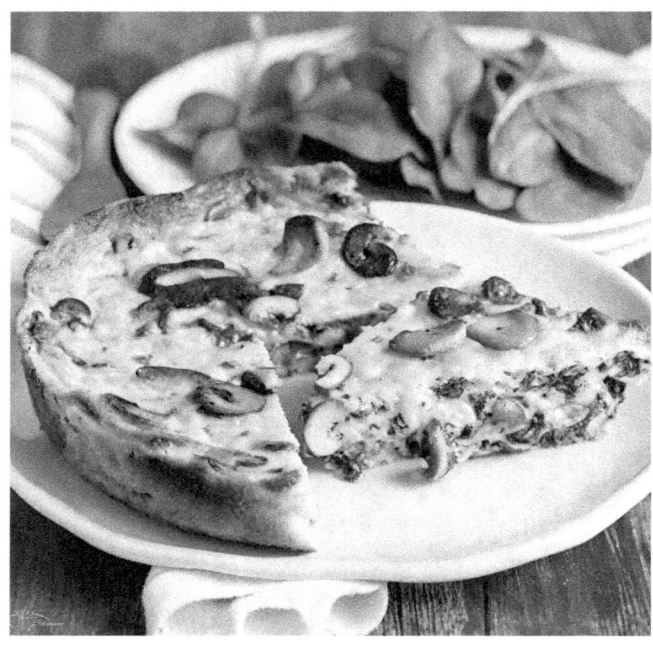

18. Kale and Sweet Potato Hash

Ingredients:
- 2 medium sweet potatoes, diced
- 1 bunch kale, chopped
- 1 onion, diced
- 2 cloves garlic, minced
- 2 tablespoons olive oil
- 1 teaspoon smoked paprika

Instructions:
1. Heat olive oil in a large skillet over medium heat.
2. Add sweet potatoes and onions, cooking until the potatoes are tender.
3. Add garlic, kale, and smoked paprika, cooking until the kale is wilted and everything is well combined.
4. Serve warm.

Nutrition Info (per serving, serves 4):
- Calories: 200
- Protein: 3 g
- Carbohydrates: 30 g
- Fat: 9 g
- Fiber: 5 g

Cooking Time: 25 minutes

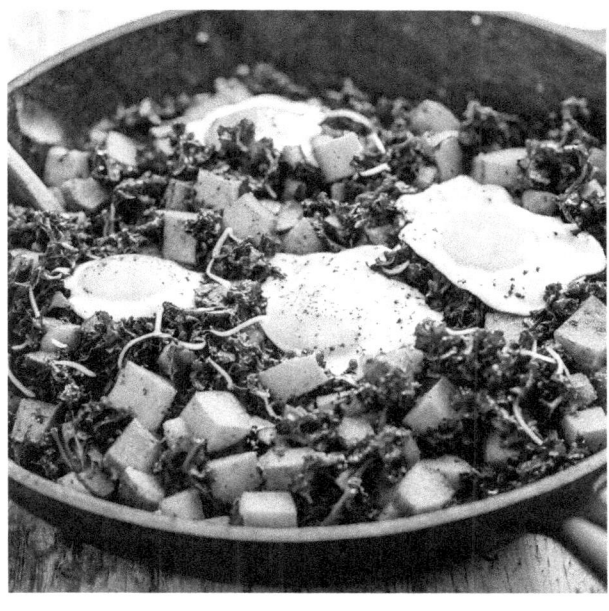

19. Apple Cinnamon Millet Bowl

Ingredients:
- 1 cup millet
- 3 cups water
- 1 apple, diced
- 1/2 teaspoon cinnamon
- 1 tablespoon honey or maple syrup
- 1/4 cup chopped walnuts

Instructions:
1. Rinse millet and cook in water until tender, about 20 minutes.
2. Stir in diced apple, cinnamon, and sweetener of choice.
3. Cook for an additional 5 minutes.
4. Serve topped with chopped walnuts.

Nutrition Info (per serving, serves 4):
- Calories: 240
- Protein: 6 g
- Carbohydrates: 46 g
- Fat: 5 g
- Fiber: 6 g

Cooking Time: 25 minutes

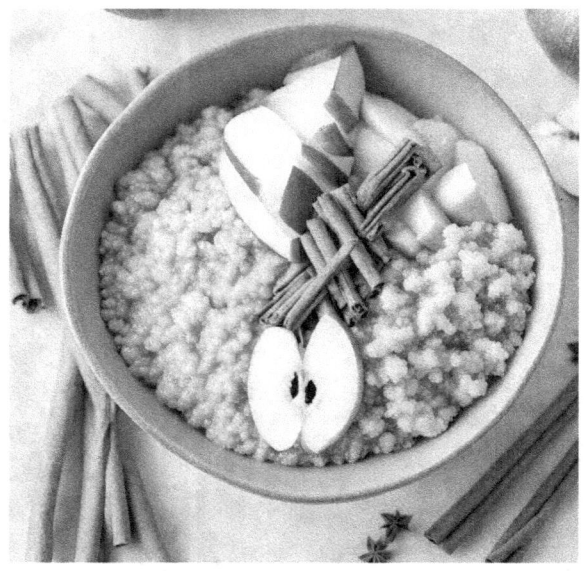

20. Sautéed Greens

Ingredients:
- 4 cups mixed greens (kale, spinach, chard)
- 2 cloves garlic, minced
- 2 tablespoons olive oil
- 1 tablespoon lemon juice

Instructions:
1. Heat olive oil in a large skillet over medium heat.
2. Add garlic and sauté for 1 minute.
3. Add greens and cook until wilted.
4. Drizzle with lemon juice before serving.

Nutrition Info (per serving, serves 4):
- Calories: 80
- Protein: 2 g
- Carbohydrates: 4 g
- Fat: 7 g
- Fiber: 2 g

Cooking Time: 10 minutes

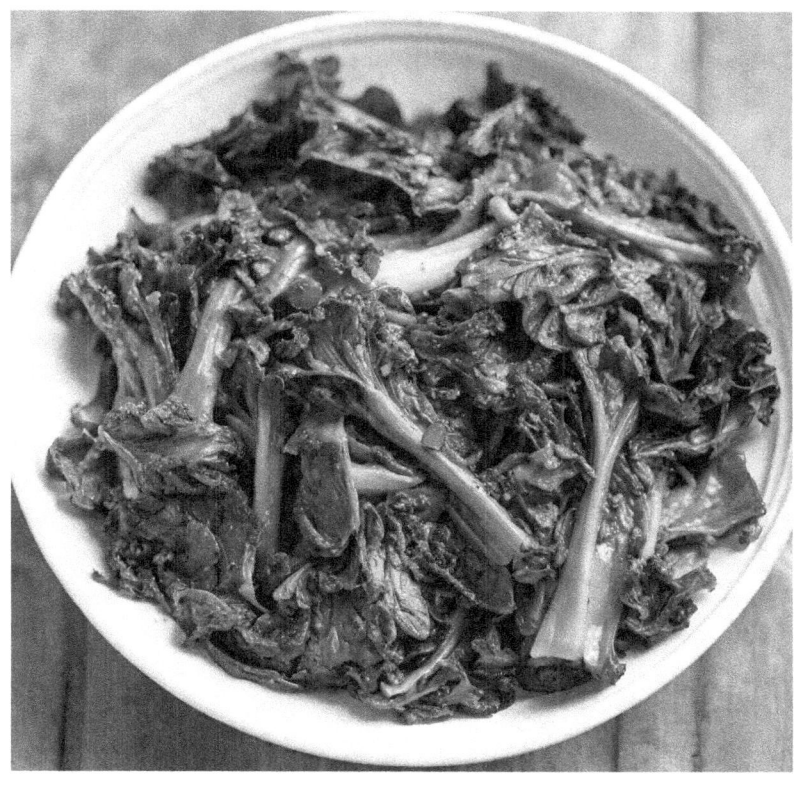

21. Polenta

Ingredients:
- 1 cup polenta (cornmeal)
- 4 cups water
- 1 tablespoon olive oil
- 1/4 cup grated Parmesan cheese (optional)

Instructions:
1. Bring water to a boil in a saucepan.
2. Gradually whisk in polenta and reduce heat to low.
3. Cook, stirring frequently, until polenta is thick and creamy, about 30-40 minutes.
4. Stir in olive oil and Parmesan cheese if using before serving.

Nutrition Info (per serving, serves 4):
- Calories: 220
- Protein: 4 g
- Carbohydrates: 31 g
- Fat: 9 g (including cheese)
- Fiber: 1 g

Cooking Time: 40 minutes

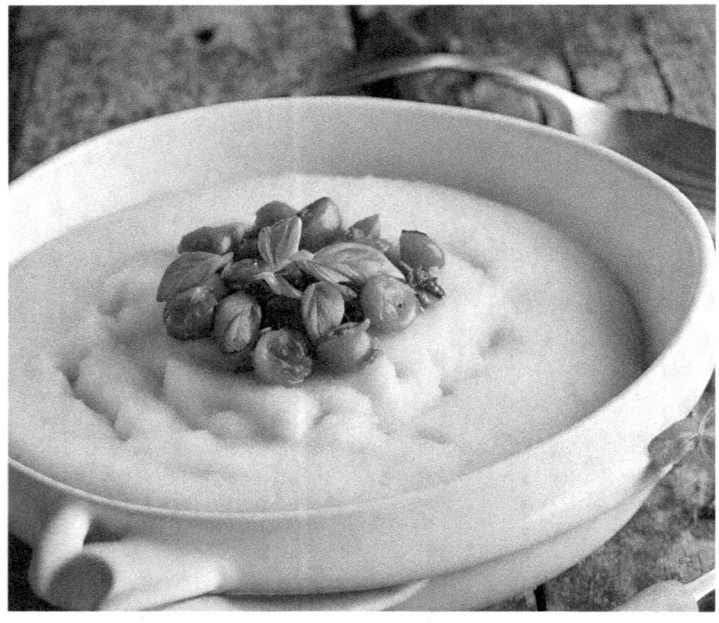

22. Carrot Cake Oatmeal

Ingredients:
- 1 cup rolled oats
- 2 cups water
- 1 large carrot, grated
- 1/2 teaspoon cinnamon
- 1/4 teaspoon nutmeg
- 2 tablespoons raisins
- 1 tablespoon maple syrup
- 1/4 cup chopped walnuts

Instructions:
1. Bring water to a boil, then add oats and reduce heat to simmer.
2. Stir in grated carrot, cinnamon, nutmeg, and raisins.
3. Cook until oats are soft and creamy, about 10 minutes.
4. Stir in maple syrup and serve topped with walnuts.

Nutrition Info (per serving, serves 2):
- Calories: 350
- Protein: 8 g
- Carbohydrates: 60 g
- Fat: 11 g
- Fiber: 8 g

Cooking Time: 15 minutes

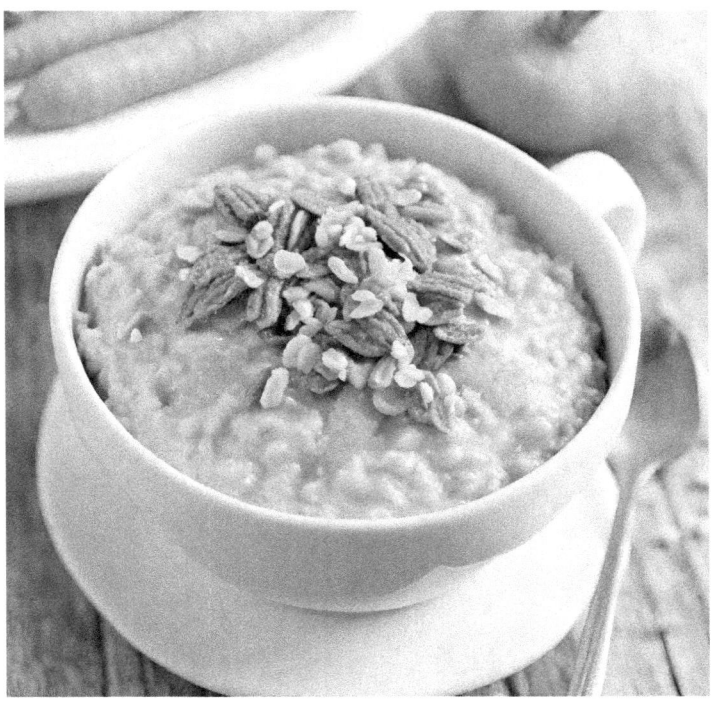

Poultry Recipes

1. Grilled Chicken Salad
Ingredients:
- 2 boneless, skinless chicken breasts
- 1 tablespoon olive oil
- 1 teaspoon garlic powder
- 1 teaspoon dried oregano
- 4 cups mixed salad greens
- 1 cucumber, sliced
- 1/2 red onion, thinly sliced
- 1/4 cup sliced almonds
- 1/4 cup balsamic vinaigrette

Instructions:
1. Preheat the grill to medium-high heat.
2. Rub chicken breasts with olive oil, garlic powder, and oregano.
3. Grill chicken for 6-7 minutes on each side until fully cooked and juices run clear.
4. Let chicken rest for a few minutes, then slice.
5. Toss salad greens, cucumber, red onion, and grilled chicken in a large bowl.
6. Drizzle with balsamic vinaigrette and sprinkle with sliced almonds.

Nutrition Info (per serving, serves 4):
- Calories: 230
- Protein: 26 g
- Carbohydrates: 9 g
- Fat: 11 g
- Fiber: 3 g

Cooking Time: 20 minutes

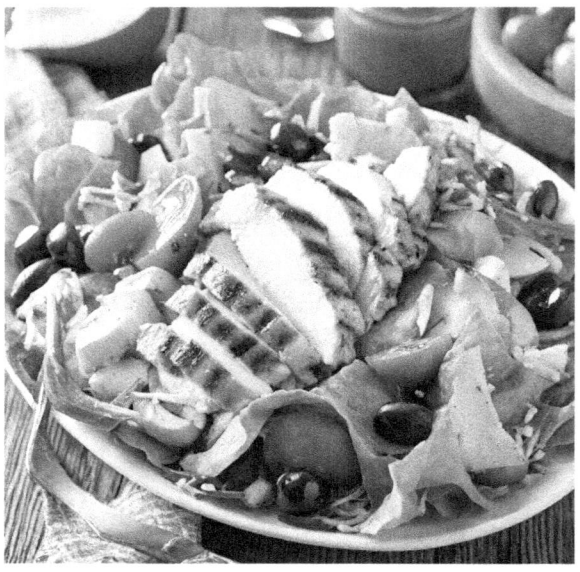

2. Turkey Meatballs

Ingredients:
- 1 pound ground turkey
- 1 egg
- 1/4 cup breadcrumbs (gluten-free if needed)
- 1/4 cup grated carrot
- 1/4 cup finely chopped onion
- 1 teaspoon dried basil
- 1 teaspoon dried parsley
- 2 tablespoons olive oil

Instructions:
1. Preheat the oven to 375°F (190°C).
2. In a bowl, combine ground turkey, egg, breadcrumbs, carrot, onion, basil, and parsley.
3. Mix well and shape into 1-inch meatballs.
4. Place meatballs on a baking sheet and drizzle with olive oil.
5. Bake for 25-30 minutes until cooked through and lightly browned.

Nutrition Info (per serving, serves 4):
- Calories: 240
- Protein: 27 g
- Carbohydrates: 7 g
- Fat: 12 g
- Fiber: 1 g

Cooking Time: 30 minutes

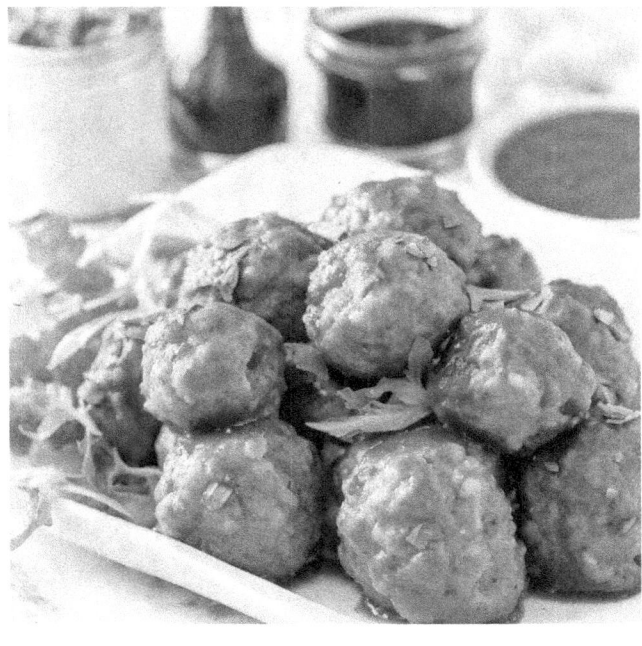

3. Chicken Stir-Fry

Ingredients:
- 1 pound chicken breast, thinly sliced
- 2 tablespoons olive oil
- 1 bell pepper, sliced
- 1 carrot, julienned
- 1 zucchini, sliced
- 1/2 cup broccoli florets
- 2 cloves garlic, minced
- 1/4 cup soy sauce (low sodium)
- 1 tablespoon sesame oil
- 1 teaspoon ginger, grated

Instructions:
1. Heat olive oil in a large skillet over medium-high heat.
2. Add chicken slices and cook until browned and nearly cooked through.
3. Add garlic, bell pepper, carrot, zucchini, and broccoli. Stir-fry until vegetables are tender.
4. Pour in soy sauce, sesame oil, and ginger. Cook for another 2-3 minutes, stirring to combine flavors.
5. Serve hot.

Nutrition Info (per serving, serves 4):
- Calories: 280
- Protein: 28 g
- Carbohydrates: 9 g
- Fat: 15 g
- Fiber: 2 g

Cooking Time: 20 minutes

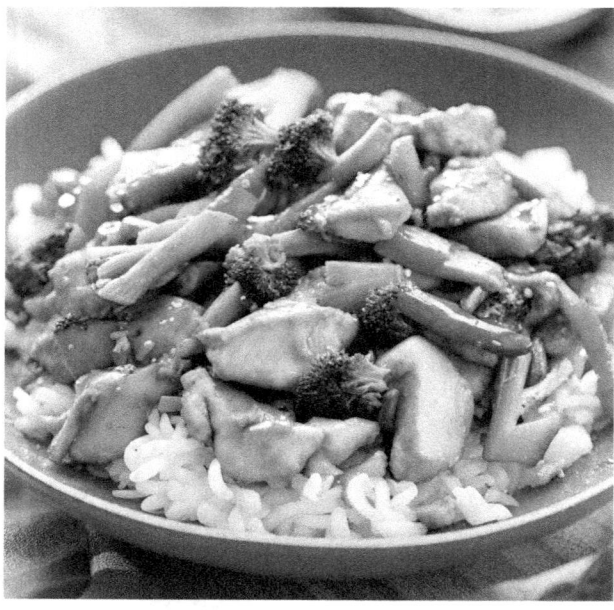

4. Roasted Turkey Breast

Ingredients:
- 1 turkey breast (about 3 pounds)
- 2 tablespoons olive oil
- 1 teaspoon thyme
- 1 teaspoon rosemary
- 1/2 lemon, juiced

Instructions:
1. Preheat the oven to 350°F (175°C).
2. Rub the turkey breast with olive oil, thyme, rosemary, and lemon juice.
3. Place in a roasting pan and bake for 1-1.5 hours, or until the turkey reaches an internal temperature of 165°F (74°C).
4. Let rest before slicing.

Nutrition Info (per serving, serves 6):
- Calories: 210
- Protein: 35 g
- Carbohydrates: 0 g
- Fat: 7 g
- Fiber: 0 g

Cooking Time: 90 minutes

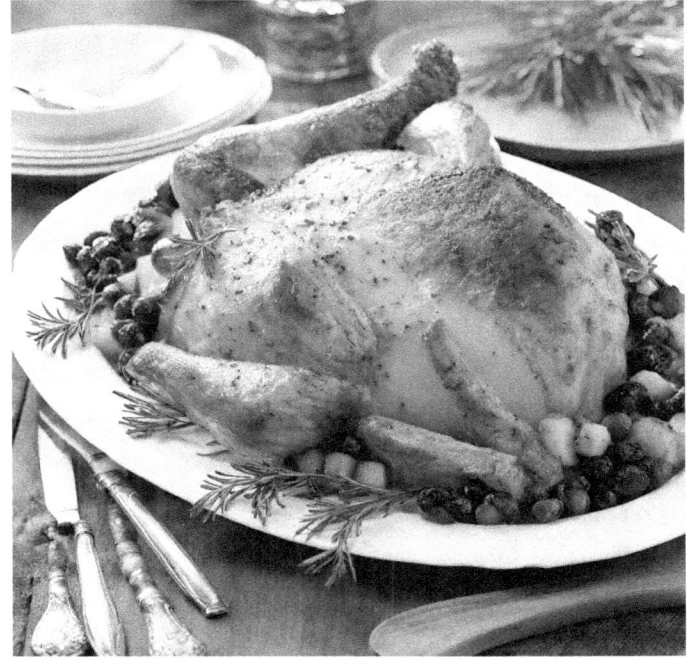

5. Chicken Soup

Ingredients:
- 1 pound chicken breast, cubed
- 1 tablespoon olive oil
- 1 onion, chopped
- 2 carrots, sliced
- 2 celery stalks, sliced
- 6 cups chicken broth (low sodium)
- 1 teaspoon dried parsley
- 1/2 teaspoon thyme

Instructions:
1. Heat olive oil in a large pot over medium heat.
2. Add chicken and cook until browned.
3. Add onion, carrots, and celery and cook for a few minutes until softened.
4. Pour in chicken broth and bring to a boil.
5. Reduce heat and simmer for 20 minutes.
6. Add parsley and thyme and cook for an additional 10 minutes.
7. Serve hot.

Nutrition Info (per serving, serves 4):
- Calories: 210
- Protein: 27 g
- Carbohydrates: 9 g
- Fat: 7 g
- Fiber: 2 g

Cooking Time: 40 minutes

6. Baked Chicken with Herbs

Ingredients:
- 4 chicken thighs (bone-in, skin-on)
- 1 tablespoon olive oil
- 1 teaspoon dried rosemary
- 1 teaspoon dried thyme
- 1 lemon, sliced

Instructions:
1. Preheat the oven to 400°F (200°C).
2. Rub chicken thighs with olive oil, rosemary, and thyme.
3. Place lemon slices under and on top of the chicken in a baking dish.
4. Bake for 35-40 minutes, or until the chicken is golden and cooked through.

Nutrition Info (per serving, serves 4):
- Calories: 300
- Protein: 24 g
- Carbohydrates: 3 g
- Fat: 22 g
- Fiber: 1 g

Cooking Time: 40 minutes

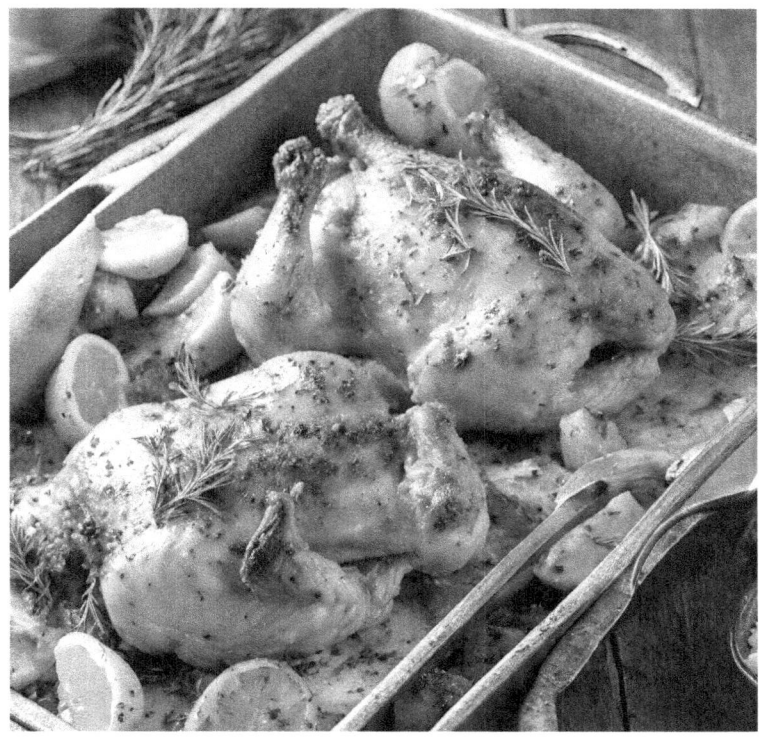

7. Chicken Curry

Ingredients:
- 1 pound chicken breast, cubed
- 2 tablespoons olive oil
- 1 onion, chopped
- 2 cloves garlic, minced
- 1 tablespoon grated ginger
- 1 tablespoon curry powder
- 1 can (14 oz) coconut milk
- 1 cup diced tomatoes
- 1/2 cup frozen peas
- Fresh cilantro, chopped for garnish

Instructions:
1. Heat olive oil in a skillet over medium heat.
2. Sauté onion, garlic, and ginger until onion is translucent.
3. Add chicken and curry powder, cook until chicken is browned.
4. Pour in coconut milk and tomatoes, bring to a simmer.
5. Reduce heat and cook for 20 minutes.
6. Stir in peas and cook for another 5 minutes.
7. Garnish with cilantro before serving.

Nutrition Info (per serving, serves 4):
- Calories: 330
- Protein: 25 g
- Carbohydrates: 15 g
- Fat: 20 g
- Fiber: 3 g

Cooking Time: 35 minutes

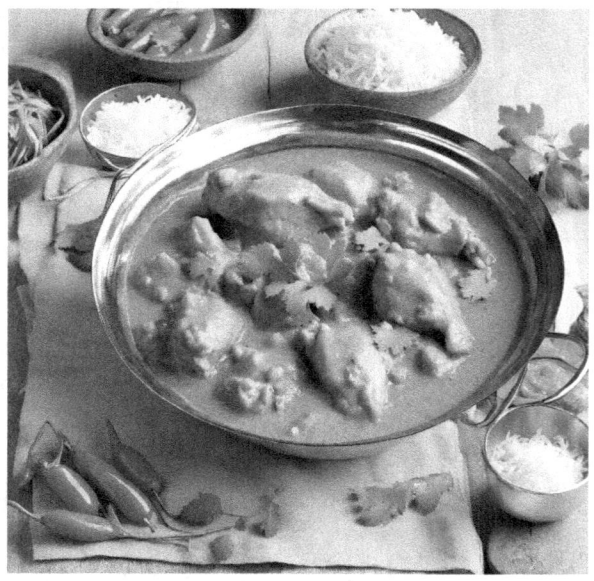

8. Poached Chicken Breast

Ingredients:
- 4 chicken breasts
- 4 cups chicken broth
- 1 onion, quartered
- 2 cloves garlic, smashed
- 1 lemon, sliced
- Fresh herbs (parsley, thyme)

Instructions:
1. In a large pot, bring chicken broth to a simmer with onion, garlic, lemon, and herbs.
2. Add chicken breasts and ensure they are submerged.
3. Simmer gently for 15-20 minutes until chicken is cooked through.
4. Remove chicken and slice for serving.

Nutrition Info (per serving, serves 4):
- Calories: 170
- Protein: 26 g
- Carbohydrates: 3 g
- Fat: 6 g
- Fiber: 0 g

Cooking Time: 25 minutes

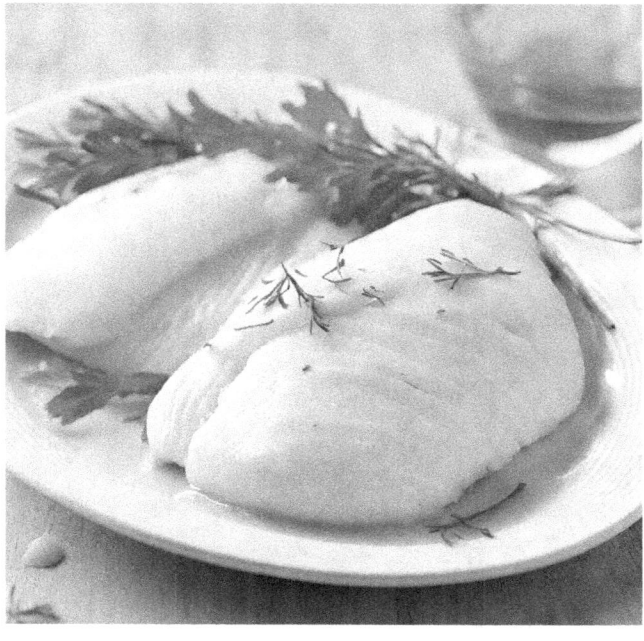

9. Turkey Stuffed Bell Peppers

Ingredients:
- 4 bell peppers, tops cut off and seeds removed
- 1 pound ground turkey
- 1 cup cooked quinoa
- 1 cup chopped spinach
- 1 onion, chopped
- 1 clove garlic, minced
- 1 cup tomato sauce
- 1 teaspoon dried oregano
- 2 tablespoons olive oil

Instructions:
1. Preheat oven to 375°F (190°C).
2. Heat olive oil in a skillet, sauté onion and garlic until soft.
3. Add ground turkey, cook until browned.
4. Stir in quinoa, spinach, tomato sauce, and oregano.
5. Stuff mixture into bell peppers, place in a baking dish.
6. Cover with foil and bake for 30 minutes. Uncover and bake for an additional 10 minutes.

Nutrition Info (per serving, serves 4):
- Calories: 350
- Protein: 28 g
- Carbohydrates: 33 g
- Fat: 15 g
- Fiber: 6 g

Cooking Time: 50 minutes

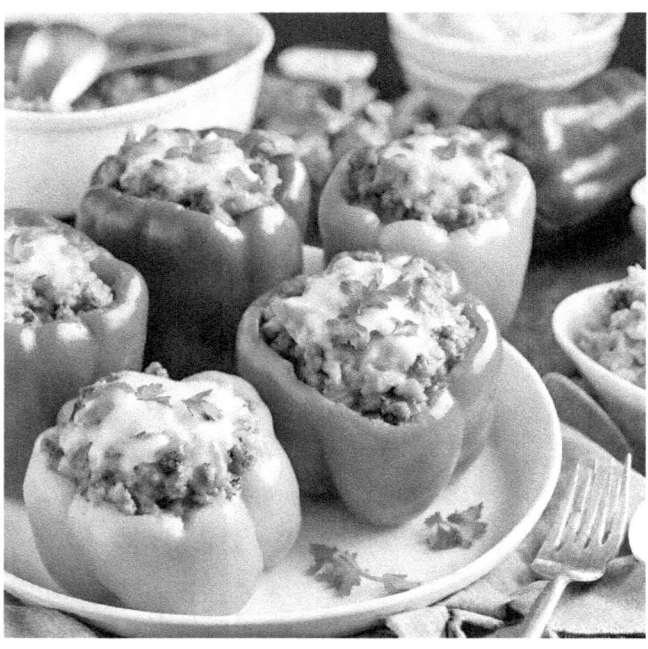

10. Baked Turkey Meatloaf

Ingredients:
- 2 pounds ground turkey
- 1 cup breadcrumbs (gluten-free if needed)
- 1 onion, finely chopped
- 1 egg, beaten
- 1/2 cup ketchup
- 1/4 cup milk (or dairy-free alternative)
- 1 teaspoon dried thyme
- 2 tablespoons Worcestershire sauce

Instructions:
1. Preheat oven to 375°F (190°C).
2. In a large bowl, mix together all ingredients until well combined.
3. Shape into a loaf on a baking tray lined with parchment paper.
4. Bake for 1 hour or until the meatloaf is cooked through.

Nutrition Info (per serving, serves 6):
- Calories: 340
- Protein: 35 g
- Carbohydrates: 20 g
- Fat: 14 g
- Fiber: 1 g

Cooking Time: 60 minutes

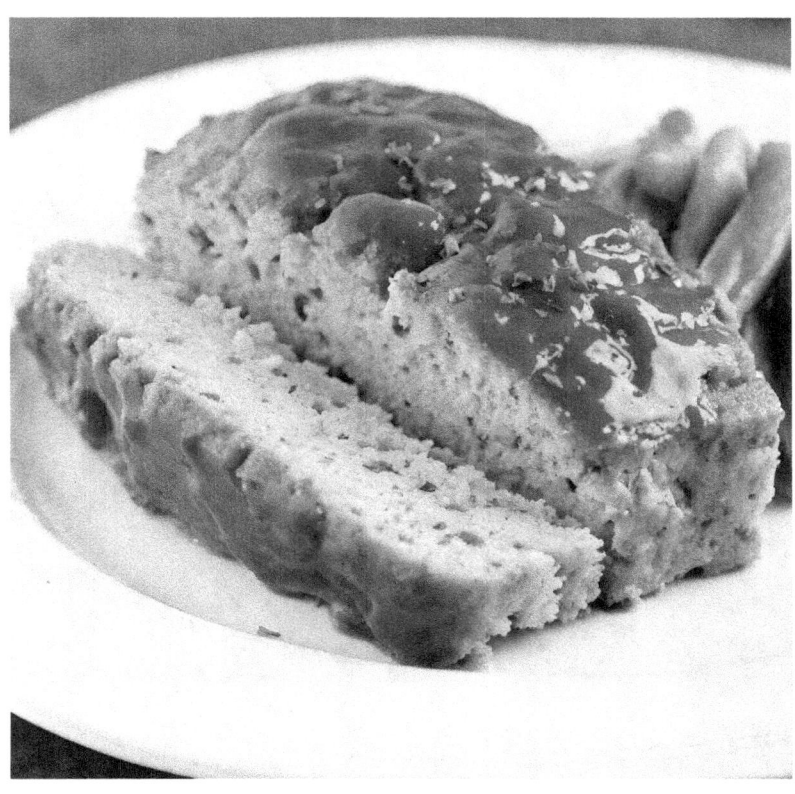

11. Chicken Vegetable Kebabs

Ingredients:
- 1 pound chicken breast, cubed
- 1 zucchini, cut into chunks
- 1 bell pepper, cut into chunks
- 1 red onion, cut into chunks
- 2 tablespoons olive oil
- 1 teaspoon garlic powder
- 1 teaspoon dried oregano
- Lemon wedges for serving

Instructions:
1. Preheat grill to medium-high heat.
2. Thread chicken and vegetables alternately onto skewers.
3. Brush with olive oil and sprinkle with garlic powder and oregano.
4. Grill for 10-15 minutes, turning occasionally, until chicken is cooked through.
5. Serve with lemon wedges.

Nutrition Info (per serving, serves 4):
- Calories: 220
- Protein: 26 g
- Carbohydrates: 10 g
- Fat: 9 g
- Fiber: 2 g

Cooking Time: 25 minutes

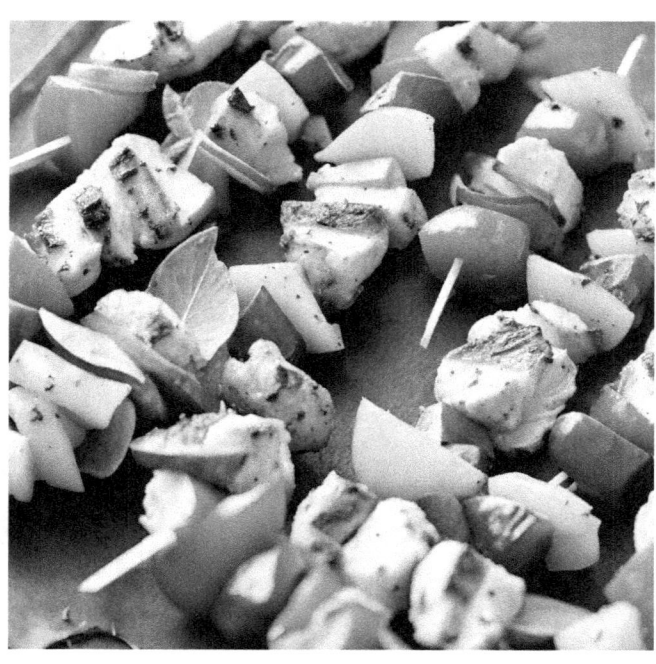

12. Stuffed Turkey Breast

Ingredients:
- 1 whole turkey breast, boneless (about 3 pounds)
- 1/2 cup dried cranberries
- 1/2 cup chopped walnuts
- 2 cups spinach, chopped
- 1 onion, finely chopped
- 2 cloves garlic, minced
- 2 tablespoons olive oil
- 1 teaspoon dried thyme

Instructions:
1. Preheat oven to 375°F (190°C).
2. In a skillet, heat 1 tablespoon olive oil over medium heat. Sauté onion and garlic until soft.
3. Add spinach, cranberries, walnuts, and thyme. Cook until spinach is wilted.
4. Butterfly the turkey breast and lay flat. Spread the stuffing mixture over the turkey.
5. Roll up the turkey breast and tie with kitchen twine. Rub the outside with the remaining olive oil.
6. Roast in the preheated oven for about 1 hour or until the internal temperature reaches 165°F (74°C).
7. Let rest before slicing.

Nutrition Info (per serving, serves 6):
- Calories: 360
- Protein: 35 g
- Carbohydrates: 15 g
- Fat: 18 g
- Fiber: 2 g

Cooking Time: 75 minutes

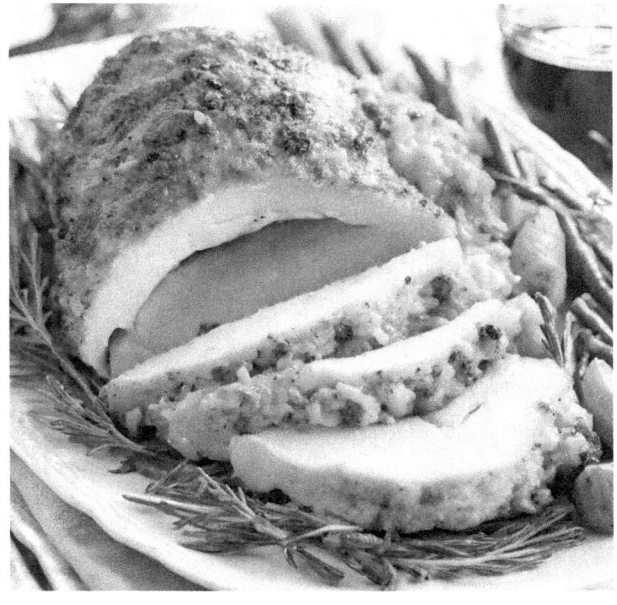

13. Chicken Paillard

Ingredients:
- 4 chicken breasts, pounded thin
- 1 lemon, juiced and zested
- 2 tablespoons olive oil
- 1/2 cup fresh parsley, chopped
- 1 clove garlic, minced

Instructions:
1. Marinate chicken breasts in lemon juice, zest, olive oil, and garlic for at least 30 minutes.
2. Heat a grill pan over medium-high heat.
3. Grill each chicken breast for about 3-4 minutes per side or until fully cooked.
4. Garnish with fresh parsley before serving.

Nutrition Info (per serving, serves 4):
- Calories: 230
- Protein: 27 g
- Carbohydrates: 3 g
- Fat: 12 g
- Fiber: 1 g

Cooking Time: 40 minutes (including marinating time)

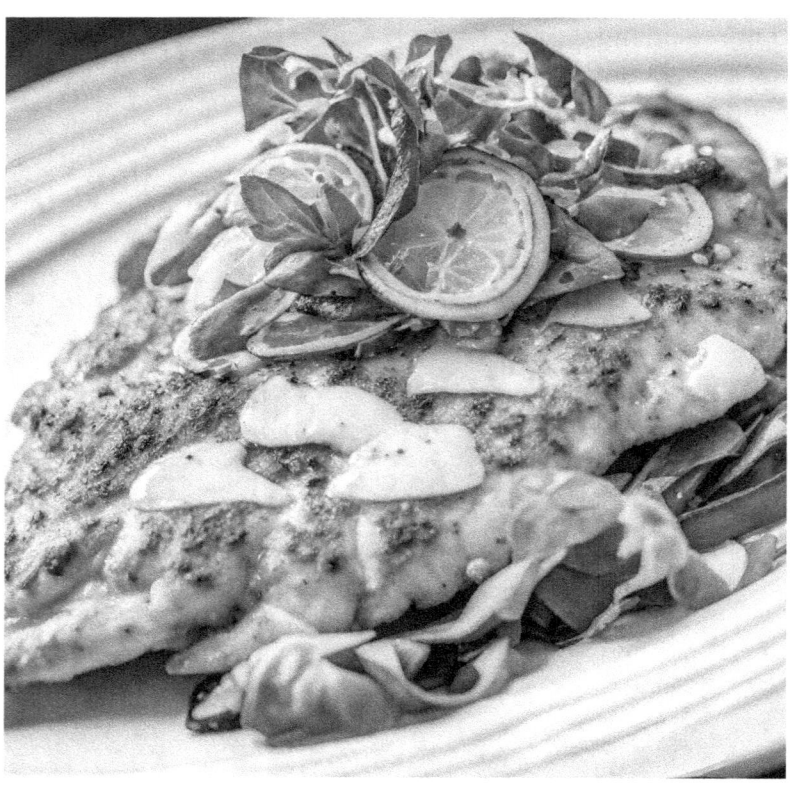

14. Turkey Skillet

Ingredients:
- 1 pound ground turkey
- 1 sweet potato, diced
- 1 bell pepper, diced
- 1 zucchini, diced
- 1 onion, chopped
- 2 tablespoons olive oil
- 1 teaspoon smoked paprika

Instructions:
1. Heat olive oil in a large skillet over medium heat.
2. Add ground turkey and cook until browned.
3. Add sweet potato, bell pepper, zucchini, and onion. Cook until vegetables are tender.
4. Stir in smoked paprika and cook for an additional 2 minutes.
5. Serve warm.

Nutrition Info (per serving, serves 4):
- Calories: 300
- Protein: 22 g
- Carbohydrates: 20 g
- Fat: 15 g
- Fiber: 3 g

Cooking Time: 30 minutes

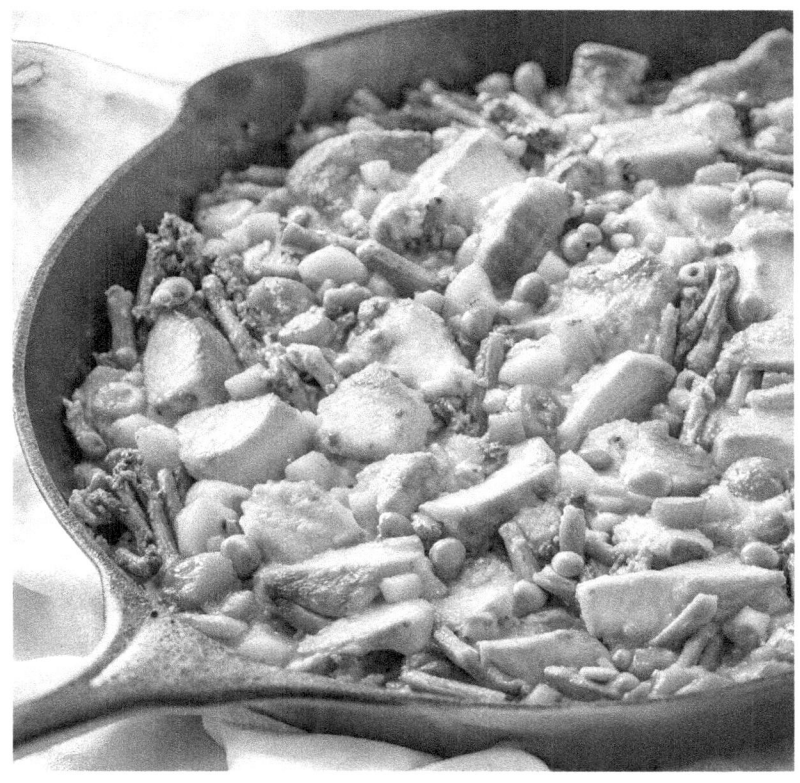

15. Chicken Piccata

Ingredients:
- 4 boneless, skinless chicken breasts, pounded thin
- 1/4 cup flour (gluten-free if necessary)
- 2 tablespoons olive oil
- 1/4 cup lemon juice
- 1/4 cup chicken broth
- 2 tablespoons capers
- 1/4 cup fresh parsley, chopped

Instructions:
1. Dredge chicken breasts in flour, shaking off excess.
2. Heat olive oil in a skillet over medium-high heat.
3. Cook chicken for 3-4 minutes on each side until golden and cooked through.
4. Remove chicken and set aside. In the same pan, add lemon juice, chicken broth, and capers.
5. Simmer for 5 minutes to reduce the sauce slightly.
6. Return chicken to the pan and coat with sauce.
7. Garnish with fresh parsley before serving.

Nutrition Info (per serving, serves 4):
- Calories: 270
- Protein: 27 g
- Carbohydrates: 10 g
- Fat: 13 g
- Fiber: 1 g

Cooking Time: 25 minutes

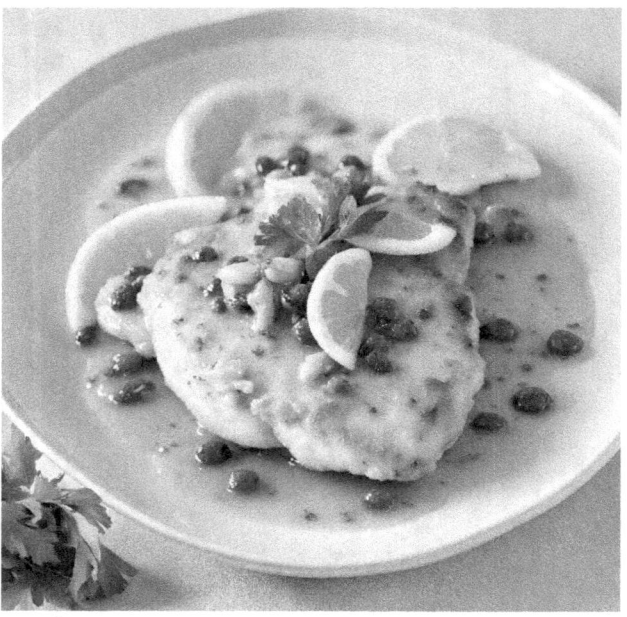

16. Roast Chicken with Thyme

Ingredients:
- 1 whole chicken (about 4 pounds)
- 2 tablespoons olive oil
- 1 tablespoon fresh thyme leaves
- 1 lemon, halved
- 1 onion, quartered
- 4 cloves garlic, smashed

Instructions:
1. Preheat oven to 400°F (200°C).
2. Rub the chicken all over with olive oil and thyme. Place lemon halves, onion quarters, and garlic inside the cavity.
3. Place the chicken in a roasting pan and roast for about 1 hour and 20 minutes, or until the juices run clear and a thermometer inserted into the thickest part of the thigh reads 165°F (74°C).
4. Let the chicken rest for 10 minutes before carving.

Nutrition Info (per serving, serves 6):
- Calories: 350
- Protein: 28 g
- Carbohydrates: 3 g
- Fat: 25 g
- Fiber: 0.5 g

Cooking Time: 90 minutes

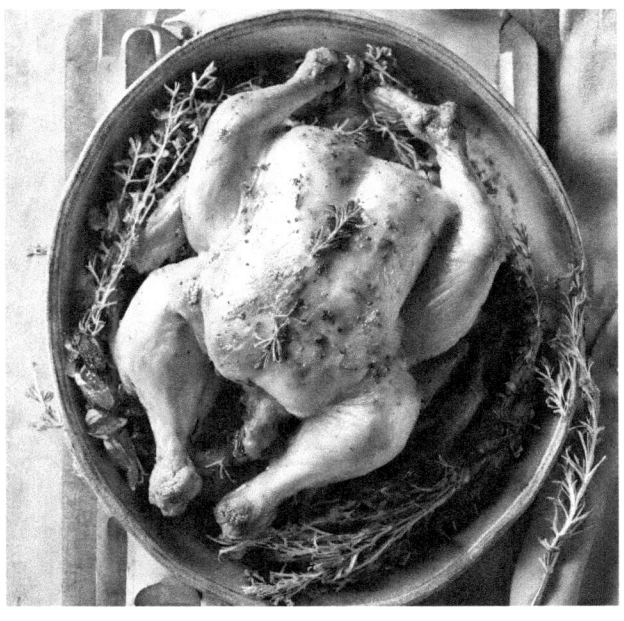

17. Turkey Soup

Ingredients:
- 1 pound cooked turkey meat, shredded
- 1 onion, chopped
- 2 carrots, sliced
- 2 celery stalks, sliced
- 6 cups chicken or turkey broth
- 1 teaspoon dried thyme
- 1 bay leaf
- 2 tablespoons olive oil

Instructions:
1. Heat olive oil in a large pot over medium heat.
2. Add onion, carrots, and celery, and sauté until vegetables are tender.
3. Add broth, turkey, thyme, and bay leaf. Bring to a boil.
4. Reduce heat and simmer for 30 minutes.
5. Remove bay leaf before serving.

Nutrition Info (per serving, serves 6):
- Calories: 180
- Protein: 20 g
- Carbohydrates: 5 g
- Fat: 9 g
- Fiber: 1 g

Cooking Time: 45 minutes

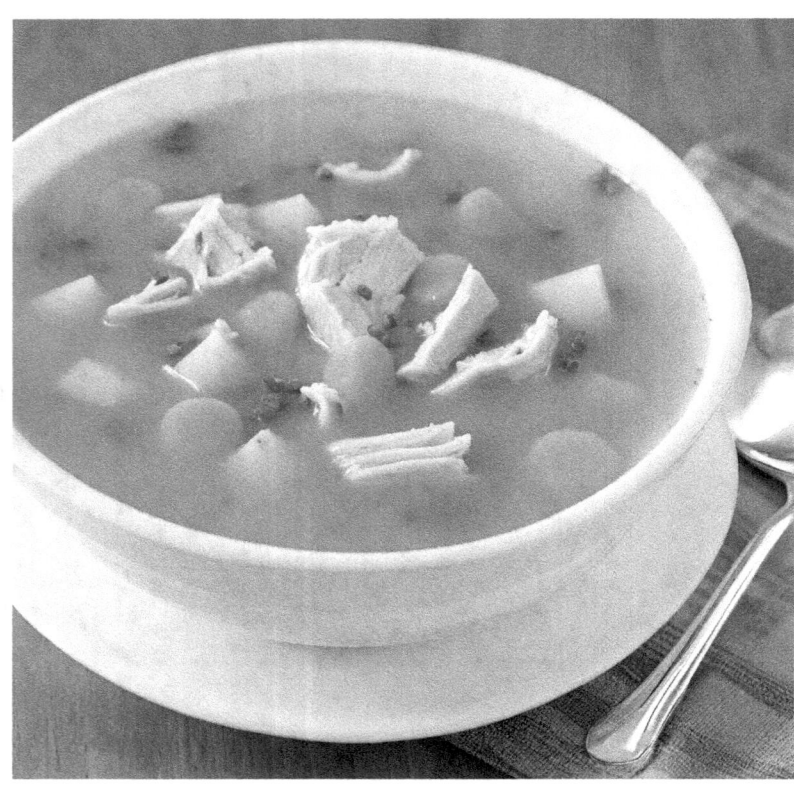

18. Chicken Caesar Salad

Ingredients:
- 2 boneless, skinless chicken breasts
- 1 tablespoon olive oil
- 4 cups romaine lettuce, chopped
- 1/2 cup Caesar dressing (low-fat)
- 1/4 cup grated Parmesan cheese
- 1 cup croutons (gluten-free if needed)

Instructions:
1. Brush chicken breasts with olive oil and grill until cooked through, about 6-7 minutes per side.
2. Let chicken rest for a few minutes, then slice thinly.
3. In a large bowl, toss lettuce with Caesar dressing, top with sliced chicken, Parmesan cheese, and croutons.

Nutrition Info (per serving, serves 4):
- Calories: 280
- Protein: 27 g
- Carbohydrates: 12 g
- Fat: 15 g
- Fiber: 2 g

Cooking Time: 20 minutes

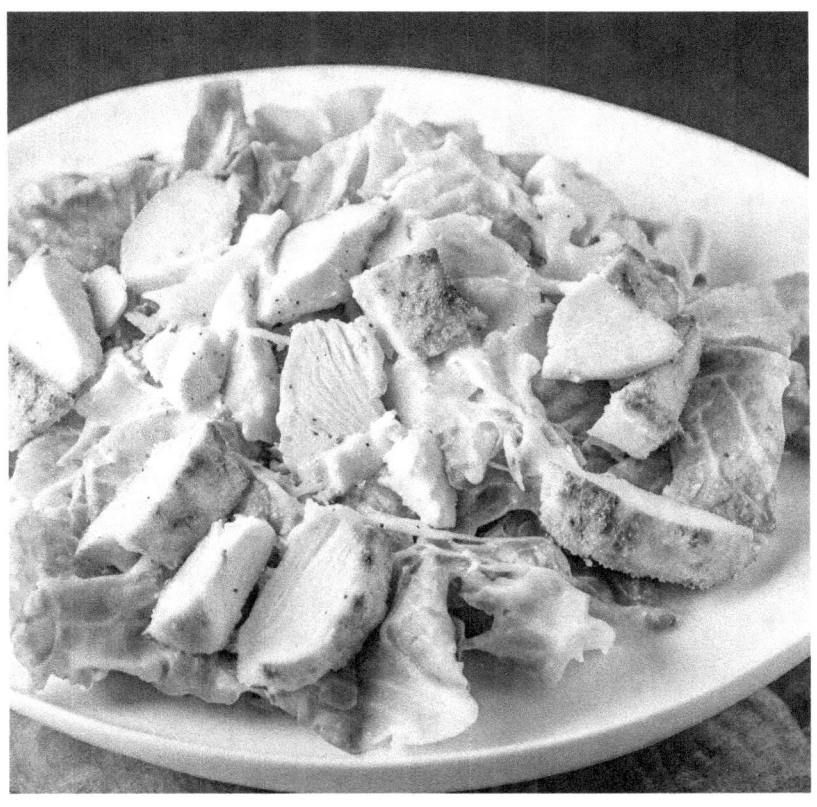

19. Slow Cooker Turkey Breast

Ingredients:
- 1 turkey breast (about 3 pounds)
- 1 onion, sliced
- 1 cup chicken broth
- 1 tablespoon olive oil
- 1 teaspoon garlic powder
- 1 teaspoon dried thyme

Instructions:
1. Place onion slices in the bottom of the slow cooker.
2. Rub turkey breast with olive oil, garlic powder, and thyme.
3. Place turkey on top of the onions and pour chicken broth around it.
4. Cover and cook on low for 6-7 hours or until the turkey is tender and reaches an internal temperature of 165°F (74°C).

Nutrition Info (per serving, serves 6):
- Calories: 220
- Protein: 35 g
- Carbohydrates: 3 g
- Fat: 8 g
- Fiber: 1 g

Cooking Time: 7 hours

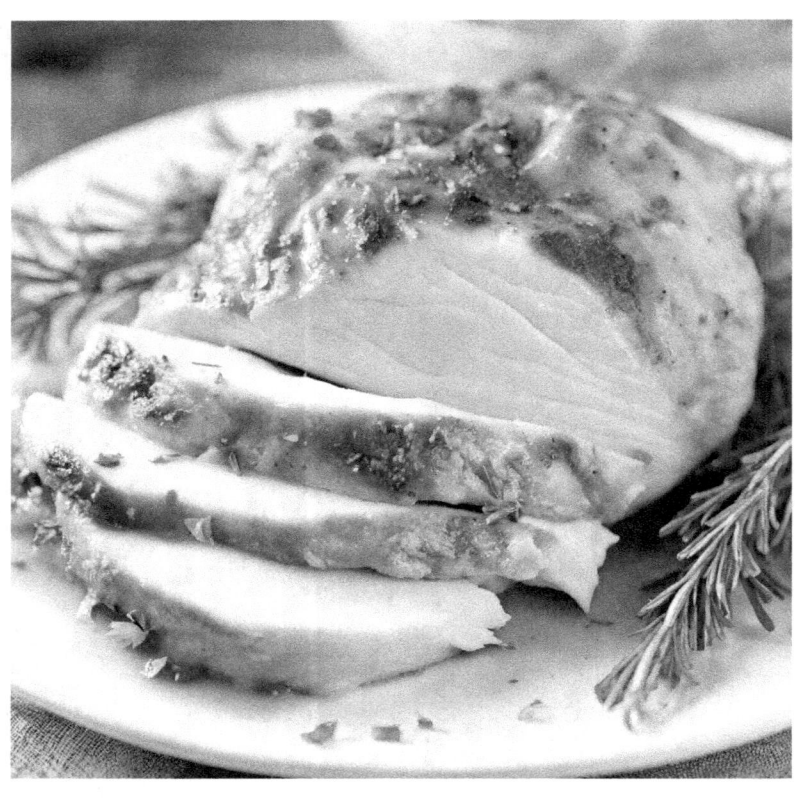

20. Turkey and Vegetable Stew

Ingredients:
- 1 pound turkey breast, cubed
- 1 onion, chopped
- 2 carrots, chopped
- 2 potatoes, cubed
- 1 celery stalk, chopped
- 4 cups chicken broth
- 1 teaspoon dried rosemary
- 2 tablespoons olive oil

Instructions:
1. Heat olive oil in a large pot over medium heat.
2. Add turkey and brown on all sides.
3. Add onion, carrots, celery, and potatoes, sautéing for a few minutes.
4. Pour in chicken broth and bring to a boil.
5. Add rosemary, reduce heat, and simmer for about 30 minutes, until vegetables are tender.

Nutrition Info (per serving, serves 4):
- Calories: 300
- Protein: 28 g
- Carbohydrates: 28 g
- Fat: 9 g
- Fiber: 4 g

Cooking Time: 45 minutes

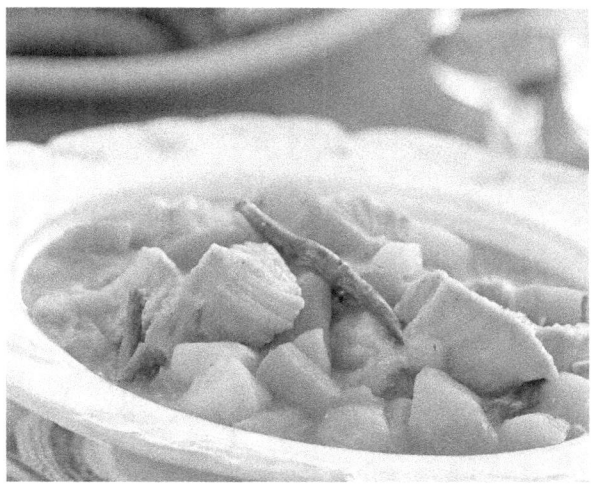

21. Grilled Chicken Caesar Wrap

Ingredients:
- 2 boneless, skinless chicken breasts
- 4 whole wheat wraps
- 2 cups romaine lettuce, shredded
- 1/2 cup Caesar dressing (low-fat)
- 1/4 cup Parmesan cheese, grated
- 1 tablespoon olive oil

Instructions:
1. Preheat the grill to medium-high heat.
2. Brush chicken breasts with olive oil and grill until cooked through, about 6-7 minutes per side.
3. Let the chicken cool slightly, then slice thinly.
4. Lay out wraps and distribute lettuce evenly among them.
5. Top each wrap with sliced chicken, a drizzle of Caesar dressing, and a sprinkle of Parmesan cheese.
6. Roll up the wraps tightly and cut in half before serving.

Nutrition Info (per serving, serves 4):
- Calories: 350
- Protein: 25 g
- Carbohydrates: 33 g
- Fat: 15 g
- Fiber: 3 g

Cooking Time: 20 minutes

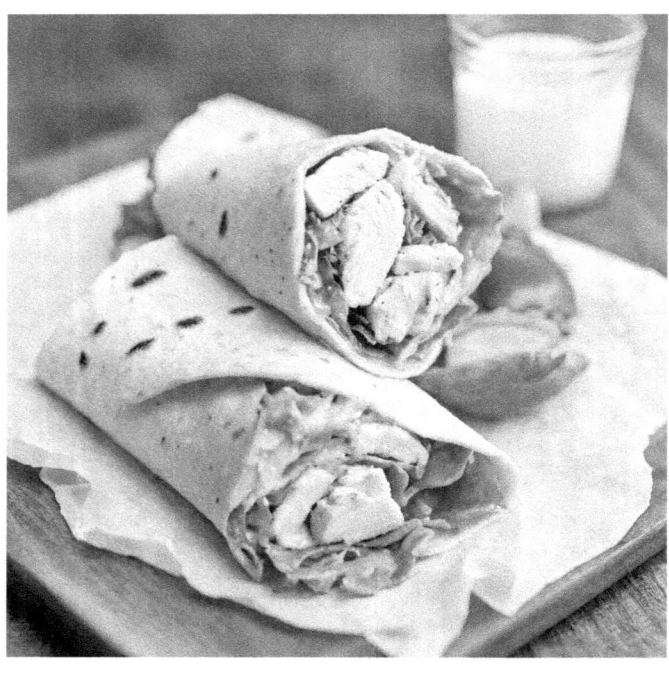

22. Lemon Garlic Turkey Cutlets

Ingredients:
- 1 pound turkey cutlets
- 2 lemons, juiced and 1 zested
- 4 cloves garlic, minced
- 2 tablespoons olive oil
- 1 tablespoon fresh parsley, chopped
- 1 teaspoon dried oregano

Instructions:
1. In a small bowl, mix lemon juice, lemon zest, garlic, olive oil, parsley, and oregano.
2. Place turkey cutlets in a shallow dish and pour the marinade over them. Marinate for at least 30 minutes.
3. Preheat a grill or skillet over medium-high heat.
4. Remove cutlets from marinade, letting excess drip off.
5. Grill or cook cutlets for about 2-3 minutes per side or until fully cooked and no longer pink in the center.
6. Serve garnished with additional fresh parsley if desired.

Nutrition Info (per serving, serves 4):
- Calories: 210
- Protein: 27 g
- Carbohydrates: 3 g
- Fat: 10 g
- Fiber: 0.5 g

Cooking Time: 40 minutes (including marinating time)

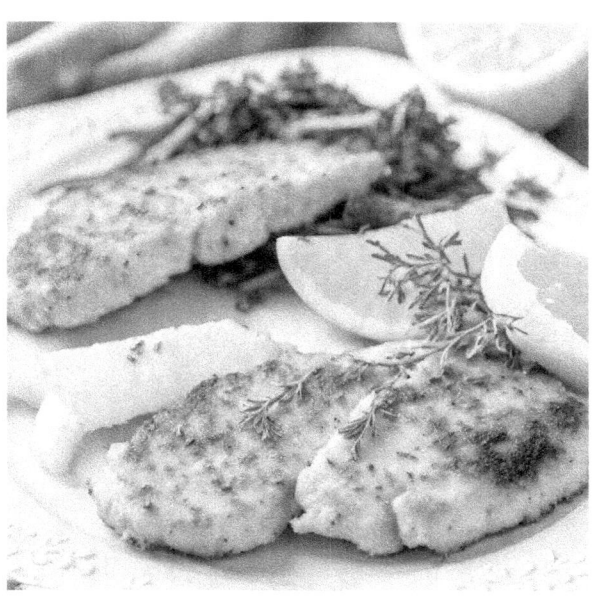

Vegetables

1. Roasted Carrot and Ginger Soup
Ingredients:
- 2 pounds carrots, peeled and chopped
- 1 onion, chopped
- 2 tablespoons fresh ginger, grated
- 4 cups vegetable broth
- 1 cup coconut milk
- 2 tablespoons olive oil
- Fresh herbs for garnish

Instructions:
1. Preheat oven to 400°F (200°C). Toss carrots and onions with olive oil and spread on a baking sheet. Roast for 25-30 minutes until carrots are tender.
2. In a large pot, combine roasted carrots and onions, ginger, and vegetable broth. Bring to a simmer.
3. Puree the mixture with an immersion blender until smooth.
4. Stir in coconut milk and heat through.
5. Serve hot, garnished with fresh herbs.

Nutrition Info (per serving, serves 6):
- Calories: 180
- Protein: 2 g
- Carbohydrates: 24 g
- Fat: 9 g
- Fiber: 6 g

Cooking Time: 45 minutes

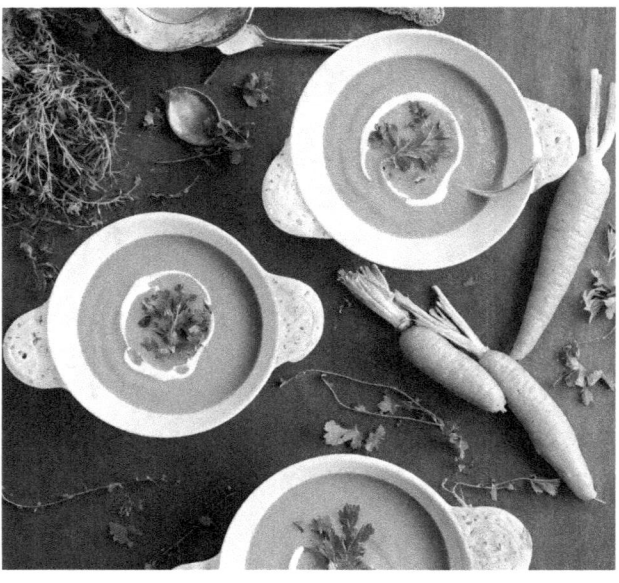

2. Sautéed Garlic Green Beans

Ingredients:
- 1 pound green beans, trimmed
- 3 cloves garlic, minced
- 2 tablespoons olive oil
- Lemon zest for garnish

Instructions:
1. Heat olive oil in a large skillet over medium heat.
2. Add garlic and sauté for about 1 minute until fragrant.
3. Add green beans and cook for 7-10 minutes, stirring occasionally, until beans are tender but still crisp.
4. Garnish with lemon zest and serve.

Nutrition Info (per serving, serves 4):
- Calories: 110
- Protein: 2 g
- Carbohydrates: 10 g
- Fat: 7 g
- Fiber: 4 g

Cooking Time: 15 minutes

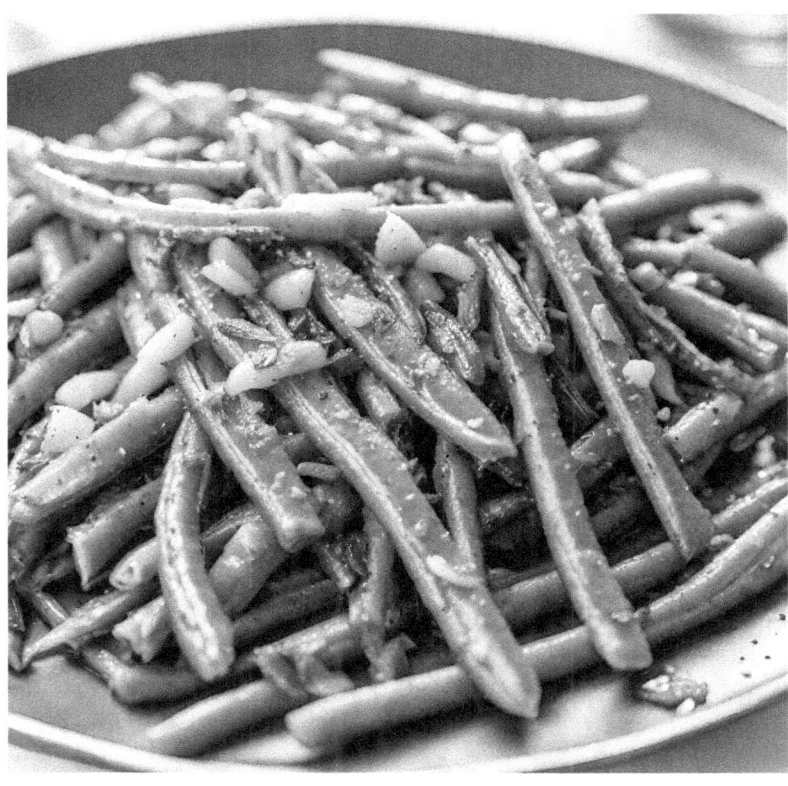

3. Spiced Roasted Butternut Squash

Ingredients:
- 1 large butternut squash, peeled and cubed
- 2 tablespoons olive oil
- 1 teaspoon cinnamon
- 1/2 teaspoon nutmeg

Instructions:
1. Preheat oven to 400°F (200°C).
2. Toss butternut squash with olive oil, cinnamon, and nutmeg.
3. Spread on a baking sheet and roast for 25-30 minutes, stirring halfway through, until tender and lightly caramelized.
4. Serve warm.

Nutrition Info (per serving, serves 4):
- Calories: 150
- Protein: 2 g
- Carbohydrates: 30 g
- Fat: 5 g
- Fiber: 6 g

Cooking Time: 30 minutes

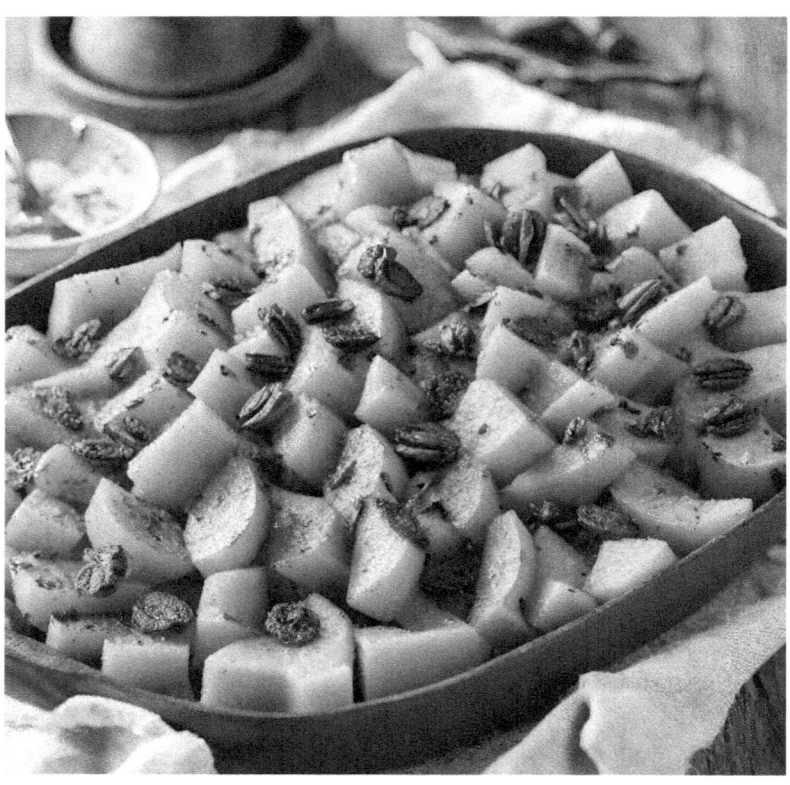

4. Grilled Asparagus with Lemon

Ingredients:
- 1 pound asparagus, trimmed
- 2 tablespoons olive oil
- 1 lemon, juiced and zested
- Fresh herbs (such as parsley or chives), chopped

Instructions:
1. Preheat grill to medium-high heat.
2. Toss asparagus with olive oil and lemon juice.
3. Grill for 4-6 minutes, turning occasionally, until tender and charred.
4. Garnish with lemon zest and fresh herbs before serving.

Nutrition Info (per serving, serves 4):
- Calories: 90
- Protein: 3 g
- Carbohydrates: 6 g
- Fat: 7 g
- Fiber: 3 g

Cooking Time: 10 minutes

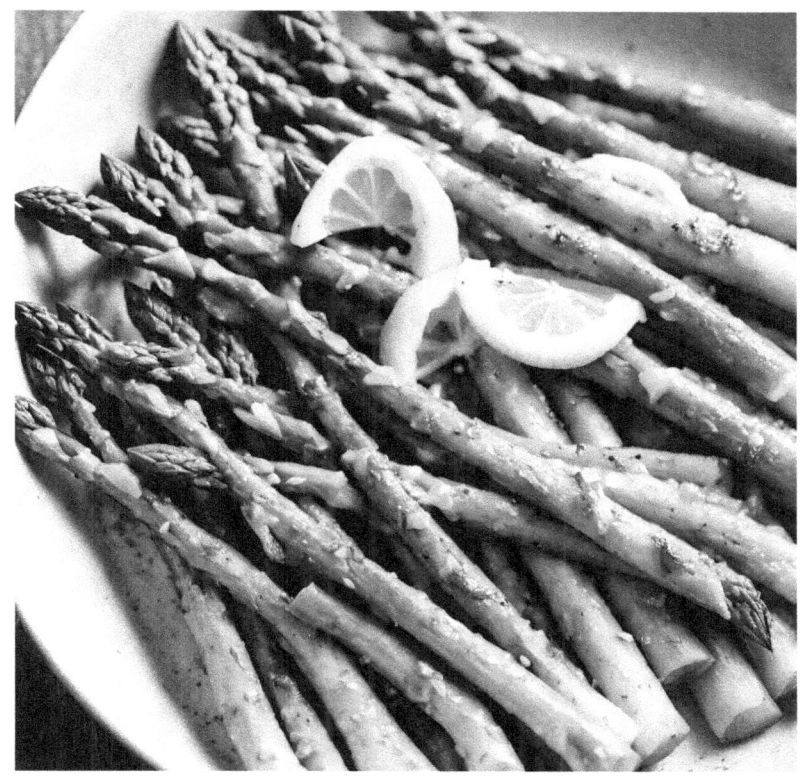

5. Zucchini Noodles with Pesto

Ingredients:
- 4 large zucchinis, spiralized into noodles
- 1 cup fresh basil leaves
- 1/2 cup grated Parmesan cheese
- 1/4 cup pine nuts
- 2 cloves garlic
- 1/2 cup olive oil
- Lemon juice to taste

Instructions:
1. In a food processor, blend basil, Parmesan, pine nuts, garlic, and olive oil until smooth to make pesto.
2. Toss zucchini noodles with pesto and a squeeze of lemon juice.
3. Serve immediately, or chill for a refreshing cold dish.

Nutrition Info (per serving, serves 4):
- Calories: 350
- Protein: 8 g
- Carbohydrates: 8 g
- Fat: 33 g
- Fiber: 2 g

Cooking Time: 15 minutes

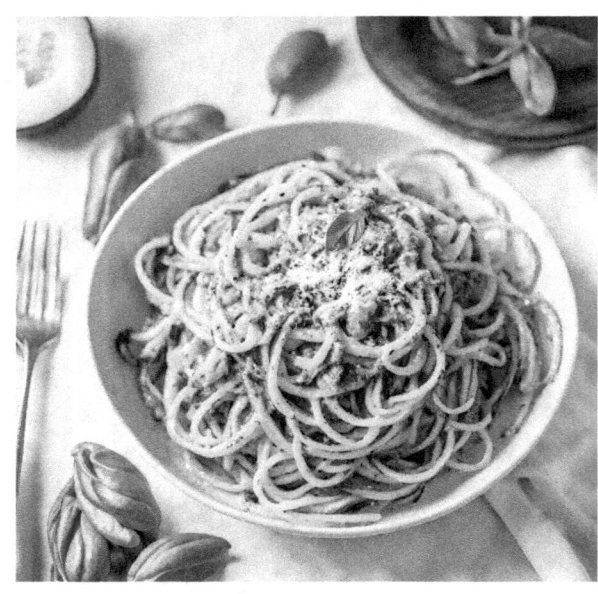

6. Kale Salad with Avocado and Almonds

Ingredients:
- 4 cups chopped kale, stems removed
- 1 ripe avocado, diced
- 1/4 cup sliced almonds, toasted
- 1 lemon, juiced
- 2 tablespoons olive oil
- 1 tablespoon honey

Instructions:
1. In a large bowl, whisk together lemon juice, olive oil, and honey.
2. Add kale to the bowl and massage the dressing into the leaves until they soften.
3. Toss in diced avocado and toasted almonds.
4. Serve chilled or at room temperature.

Nutrition Info (per serving, serves 4):
- Calories: 240
- Protein: 5 g
- Carbohydrates: 20 g
- Fat: 18 g
- Fiber: 6 g

Cooking Time: 15 minutes

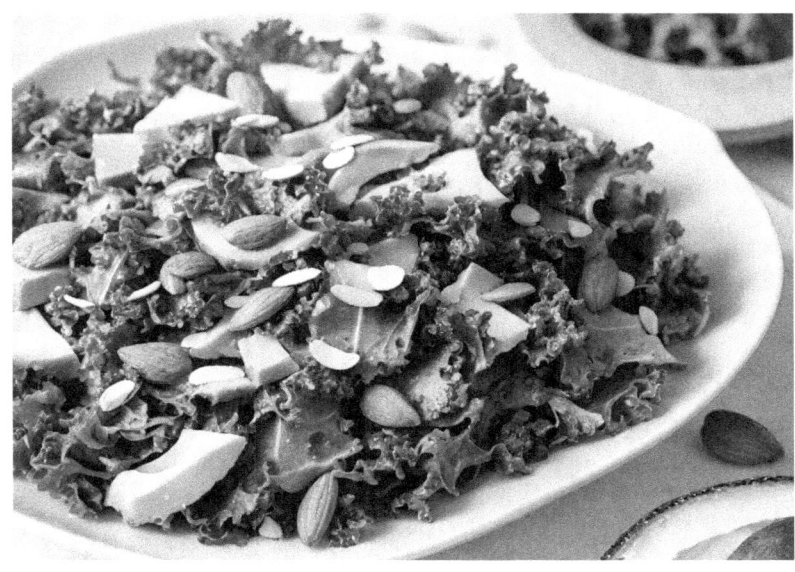

7. Spinach and Mushroom Quiche

Ingredients:
- 1 premade pie crust (gluten-free if necessary)
- 4 eggs
- 1 cup fresh spinach, chopped
- 1 cup mushrooms, sliced
- 1/2 cup milk (or almond milk)
- 1/2 cup grated cheese (optional)
- 1 tablespoon olive oil

Instructions:
1. Preheat oven to 350°F (175°C).
2. Sauté mushrooms in olive oil until they release their moisture and begin to brown.
3. In a mixing bowl, whisk together eggs and milk.
4. Stir in cooked mushrooms, spinach, and grated cheese.
5. Pour the egg mixture into the pie crust.
6. Bake for 30-35 minutes or until the center is set and the crust is golden.
7. Let cool for a few minutes before slicing.

Nutrition Info (per serving, serves 6):
- Calories: 250
- Protein: 10 g
- Carbohydrates: 15 g
- Fat: 17 g
- Fiber: 2 g

Cooking Time: 45 minutes

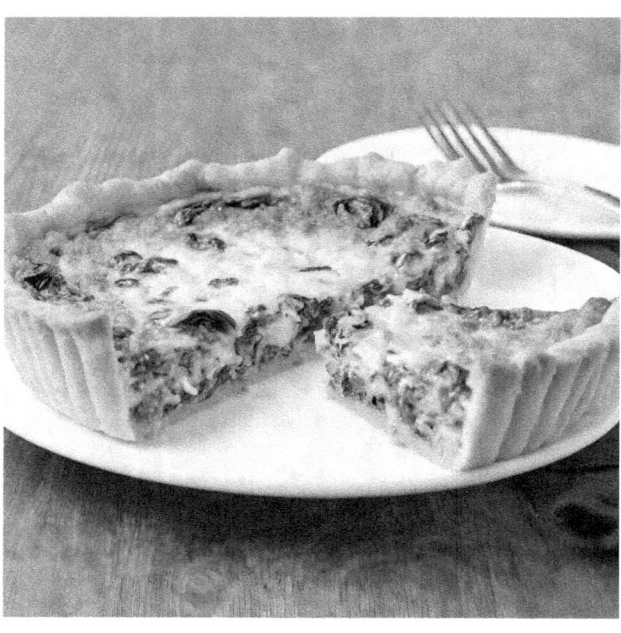

8. Beet and Carrot Slaw

Ingredients:
- 2 large beets, peeled and grated
- 2 large carrots, peeled and grated
- 1/4 cup apple cider vinegar
- 2 tablespoons olive oil
- 1 tablespoon honey
- Fresh herbs (parsley or dill), chopped

Instructions:
1. In a large bowl, whisk together apple cider vinegar, olive oil, and honey.
2. Add grated beets and carrots to the bowl and toss to coat with the dressing.
3. Garnish with fresh herbs.
4. Chill for at least 30 minutes before serving to allow flavors to meld.

Nutrition Info (per serving, serves 4):
- Calories: 140
- Protein: 2 g
- Carbohydrates: 20 g
- Fat: 7 g
- Fiber: 4 g

Cooking Time: 40 minutes (including chilling time)

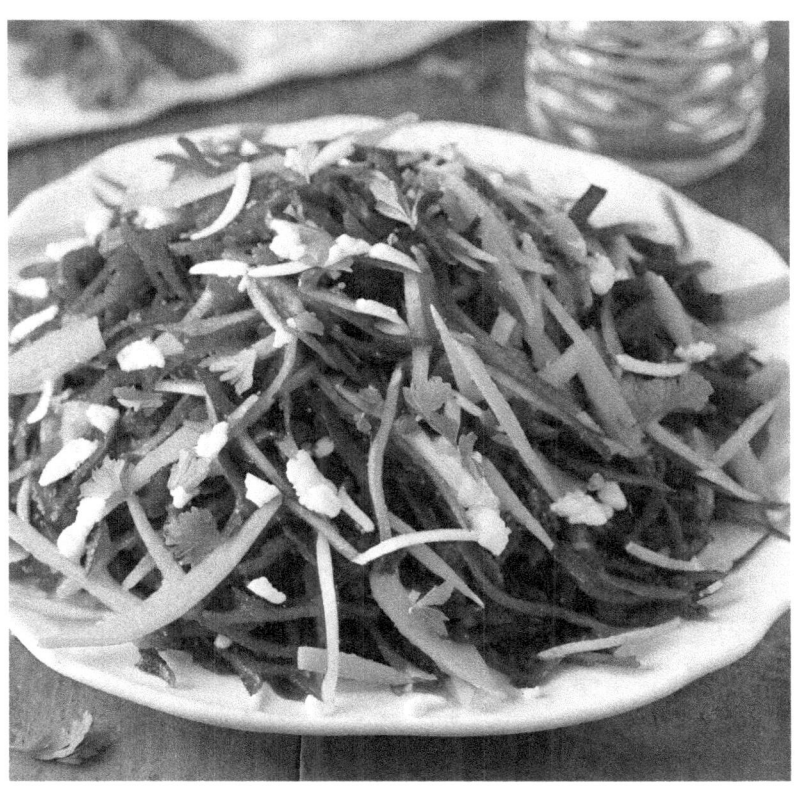

9. Grilled Eggplant with Herbs

Ingredients:
- 2 large eggplants, sliced into 1/2 inch thick rounds
- 3 tablespoons olive oil
- 2 cloves garlic, minced
- Fresh herbs (thyme, rosemary), chopped
- Lemon zest for garnish

Instructions:
1. Preheat the grill to medium-high heat.
2. Brush eggplant slices with olive oil and sprinkle with minced garlic and chopped herbs.
3. Grill for 4-5 minutes on each side until tender and grill marks appear.
4. Garnish with lemon zest before serving.

Nutrition Info (per serving, serves 4):
- Calories: 180
- Protein: 2 g
- Carbohydrates: 18 g
- Fat: 12 g
- Fiber: 6 g

Cooking Time: 20 minutes

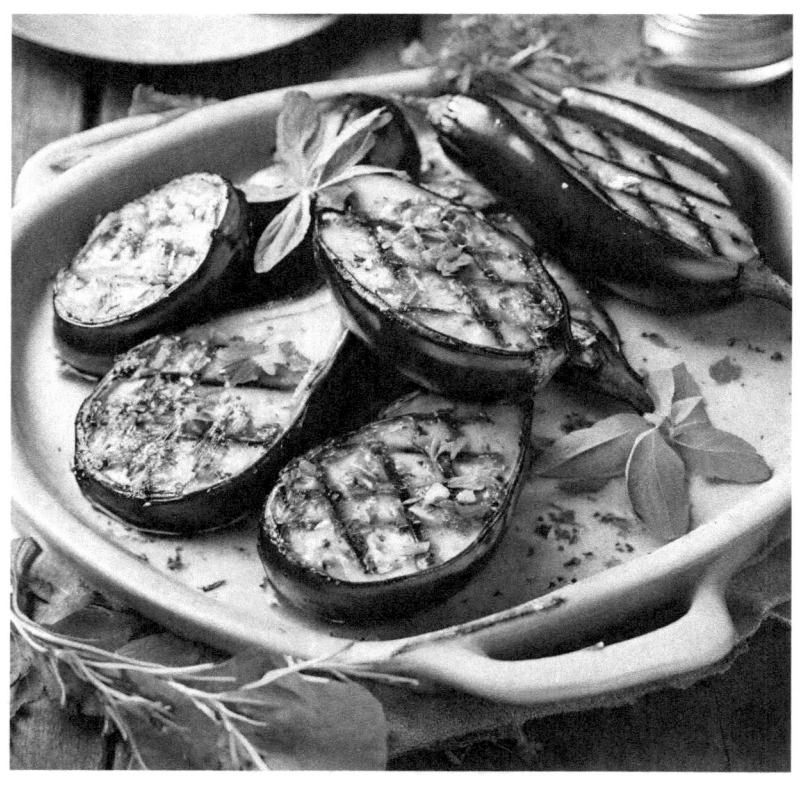

10. Vegetable Kabobs on the Grill

Ingredients:
- 1 zucchini, cut into 1-inch pieces
- 1 bell pepper, cut into 1-inch pieces
- 1 red onion, cut into wedges
- 1 cup cherry tomatoes
- 2 tablespoons olive oil
- 1 tablespoon balsamic vinegar
- Fresh herbs (basil, oregano), chopped

Instructions:
1. Preheat grill to medium-high heat.
2. Thread zucchini, bell pepper, onion, and cherry tomatoes onto skewers.
3. Whisk together olive oil and balsamic vinegar, and brush over the vegetables.
4. Grill for 10-12 minutes, turning occasionally, until vegetables are tender and slightly charred.
5. Garnish with fresh herbs before serving.

Nutrition Info (per serving, serves 4):
- Calories: 120
- Protein: 2 g
- Carbohydrates: 10 g
- Fat: 9 g
- Fiber: 2 g

Cooking Time: 25 minutes

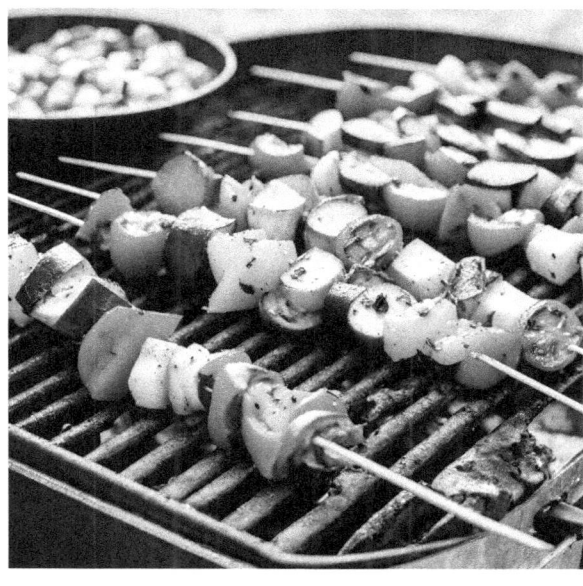

11. Spicy Stir-Fried Cabbage

Ingredients:
- 1 head of cabbage, shredded
- 2 carrots, julienned
- 1 onion, sliced
- 2 tablespoons olive oil
- 1 tablespoon apple cider vinegar
- 1 teaspoon crushed red pepper flakes
- 1 tablespoon soy sauce (low sodium)

Instructions:
1. Heat olive oil in a large skillet or wok over medium-high heat.
2. Add onion and sauté until translucent.
3. Add cabbage and carrots, stirring frequently, until the vegetables are tender and slightly caramelized, about 8-10 minutes.
4. Stir in apple cider vinegar, red pepper flakes, and soy sauce, cooking for an additional 2 minutes.
5. Serve hot.

Nutrition Info (per serving, serves 4):
- Calories: 140
- Protein: 3 g
- Carbohydrates: 18 g
- Fat: 7 g
- Fiber: 6 g

Cooking Time: 20 minutes

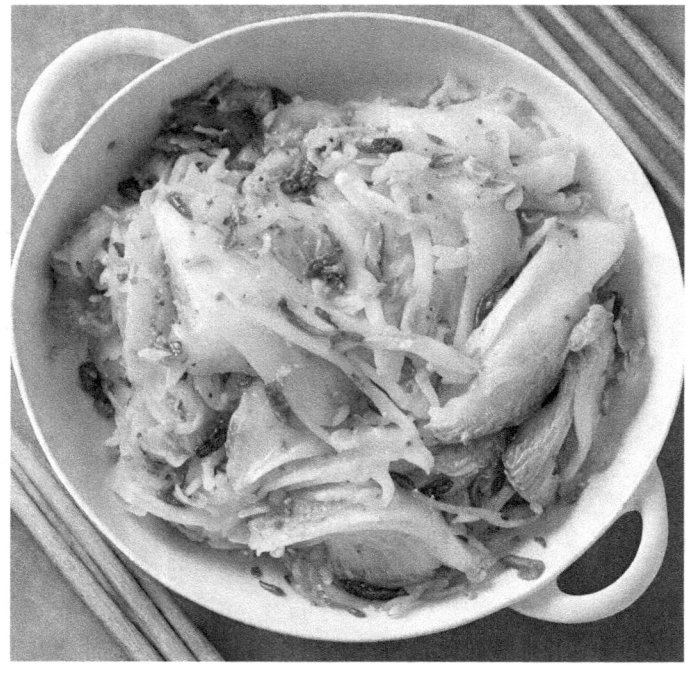

12. Watercress and Pear Salad

Ingredients:
- 4 cups watercress, trimmed
- 2 ripe pears, sliced
- 1/4 cup walnuts, toasted and chopped
- 1/4 cup blue cheese, crumbled
- 2 tablespoons olive oil
- 1 tablespoon balsamic vinegar

Instructions:
1. In a large salad bowl, combine watercress, sliced pears, walnuts, and blue cheese.
2. Whisk together olive oil and balsamic vinegar, then drizzle over the salad.
3. Toss gently to combine and serve immediately.

Nutrition Info (per serving, serves 4):
- Calories: 200
- Protein: 4 g
- Carbohydrates: 15 g
- Fat: 15 g
- Fiber: 3 g

Cooking Time: 10 minutes

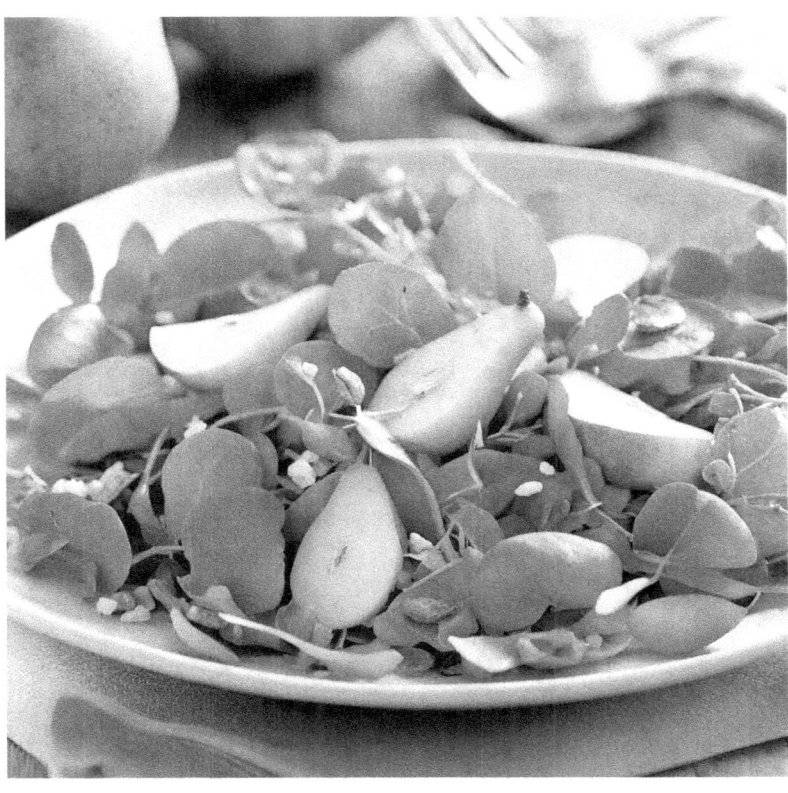

13. Balsamic Roasted Beetroot

Ingredients:
- 4 large beetroots, peeled and diced
- 2 tablespoons olive oil
- 2 tablespoons balsamic vinegar
- Fresh thyme sprigs

Instructions:
1. Preheat oven to 400°F (200°C).
2. Toss beetroots with olive oil and balsamic vinegar, and spread on a baking sheet.
3. Scatter fresh thyme sprigs over the beets.
4. Roast for 35-40 minutes, stirring occasionally, until beets are tender and caramelized.
5. Serve warm or at room temperature.

Nutrition Info (per serving, serves 4):
- Calories: 130
- Protein: 2 g
- Carbohydrates: 18 g
- Fat: 6 g
- Fiber: 5 g

Cooking Time: 40 minutes

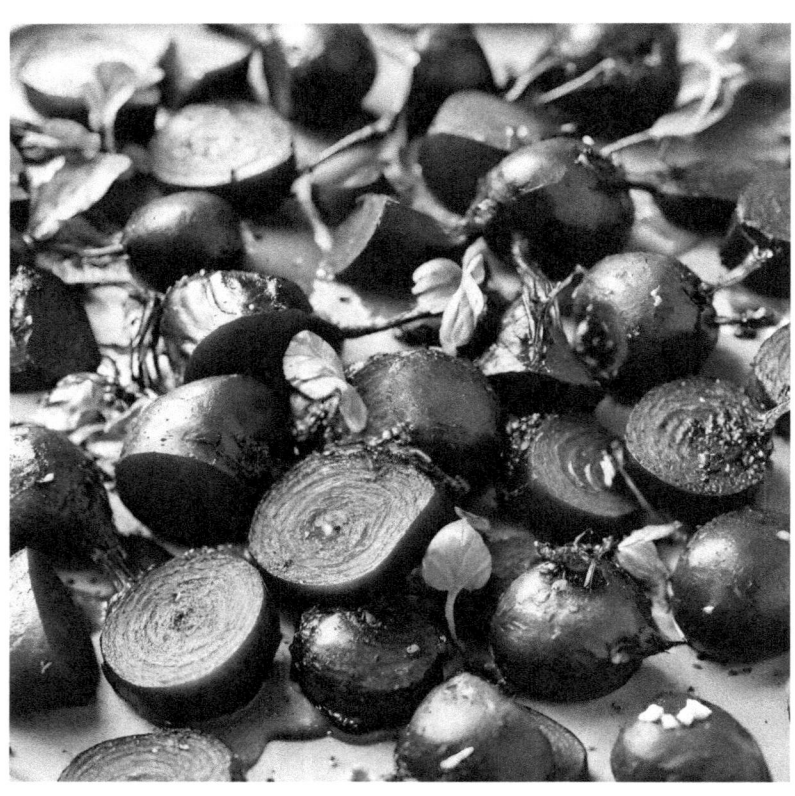

14. Swiss Chard and Lentil Stew

Ingredients:
- 1 cup lentils, rinsed
- 1 bunch Swiss chard, chopped
- 1 onion, chopped
- 2 carrots, diced
- 4 cups vegetable broth
- 2 tablespoons olive oil
- 1 teaspoon cumin
- 1 lemon, juiced

Instructions:
1. Heat olive oil in a large pot over medium heat.
2. Add onion and carrots, sauté until softened.
3. Stir in cumin and cook for 1 minute.
4. Add lentils and vegetable broth, bring to a boil.
5. Reduce heat and simmer for 20 minutes.
6. Add Swiss chard and cook until wilted, about 5 minutes.
7. Stir in lemon juice and serve hot.

Nutrition Info (per serving, serves 4):
- Calories: 250
- Protein: 12 g
- Carbohydrates: 38 g
- Fat: 7 g
- Fiber: 15 g

Cooking Time: 35 minutes

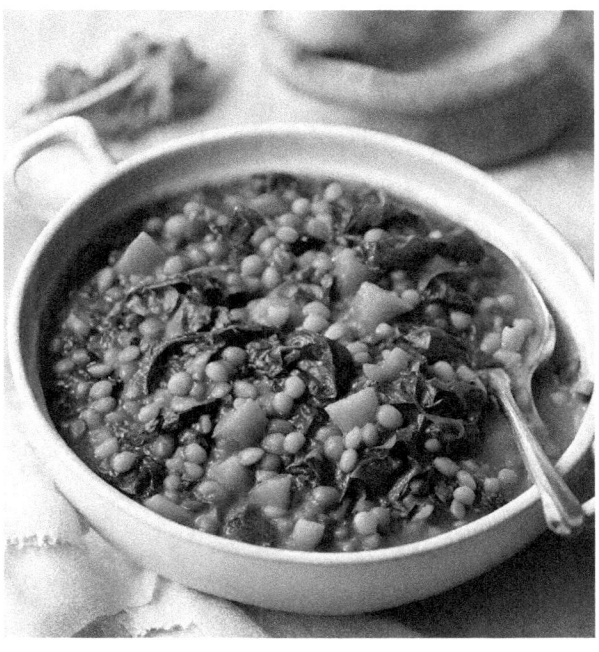

15. Herbed Potato Salad

Ingredients:
- 2 pounds small potatoes, boiled and quartered
- 1/4 cup olive oil
- 2 tablespoons lemon juice
- 1/4 cup fresh herbs (parsley, dill, chives), chopped
- 1/4 cup red onion, finely chopped

Instructions:
1. In a large bowl, whisk together olive oil and lemon juice.
2. Add boiled potatoes, fresh herbs, and red onion.
3. Toss to coat evenly.
4. Chill for at least 1 hour before serving to allow flavors to meld.

Nutrition Info (per serving, serves 4):
- Calories: 290
- Protein: 4 g
- Carbohydrates: 45 g
- Fat: 11 g
- Fiber: 6 g

Cooking Time: 1 hour 20 minutes (including cooling)

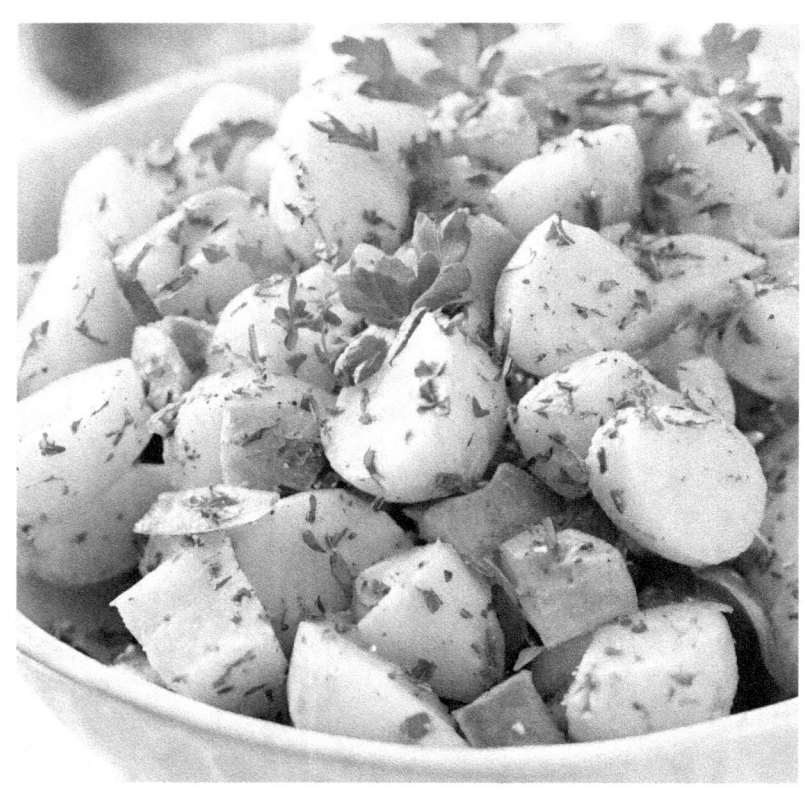

16. Asian Cucumber Salad

Ingredients:
- 2 large cucumbers, thinly sliced
- 1 red bell pepper, thinly sliced
- 1 carrot, julienned
- 1/4 cup rice vinegar
- 1 tablespoon sesame oil
- 1 tablespoon honey
- 1 teaspoon sesame seeds
- 1 tablespoon fresh cilantro, chopped

Instructions:
1. In a large bowl, combine cucumbers, red bell pepper, and carrot.
2. In a small bowl, whisk together rice vinegar, sesame oil, and honey.
3. Pour the dressing over the vegetables and toss to coat evenly.
4. Sprinkle with sesame seeds and cilantro before serving.

Nutrition Info (per serving, serves 4):
- Calories: 80
- Protein: 1 g
- Carbohydrates: 10 g
- Fat: 4.5 g
- Fiber: 2 g

Cooking Time: 10 minutes

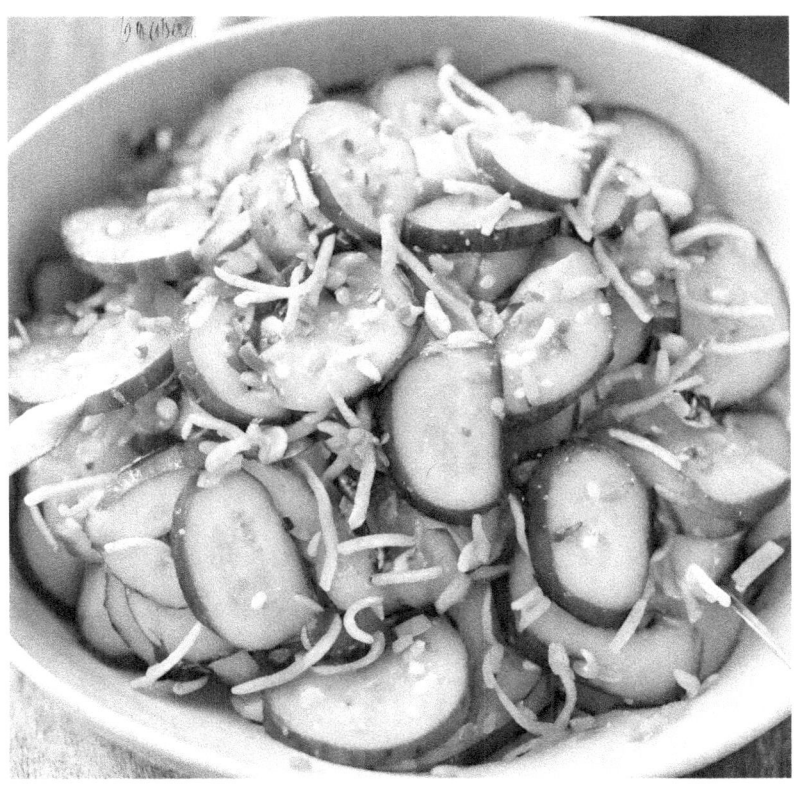

17. Sautéed Rainbow Chard with Garlic

Ingredients:
- 1 bunch rainbow chard, stems and leaves separated and chopped
- 3 cloves garlic, minced
- 2 tablespoons olive oil
- 1 tablespoon lemon juice

Instructions:
1. Heat olive oil in a large skillet over medium heat.
2. Add garlic and chard stems, sautéing until stems are tender, about 5 minutes.
3. Add chard leaves and cook until wilted, about 2-3 minutes.
4. Drizzle with lemon juice and serve immediately.

Nutrition Info (per serving, serves 4):
- Calories: 90
- Protein: 2 g
- Carbohydrates: 6 g
- Fat: 7 g
- Fiber: 2 g

Cooking Time: 10 minutes

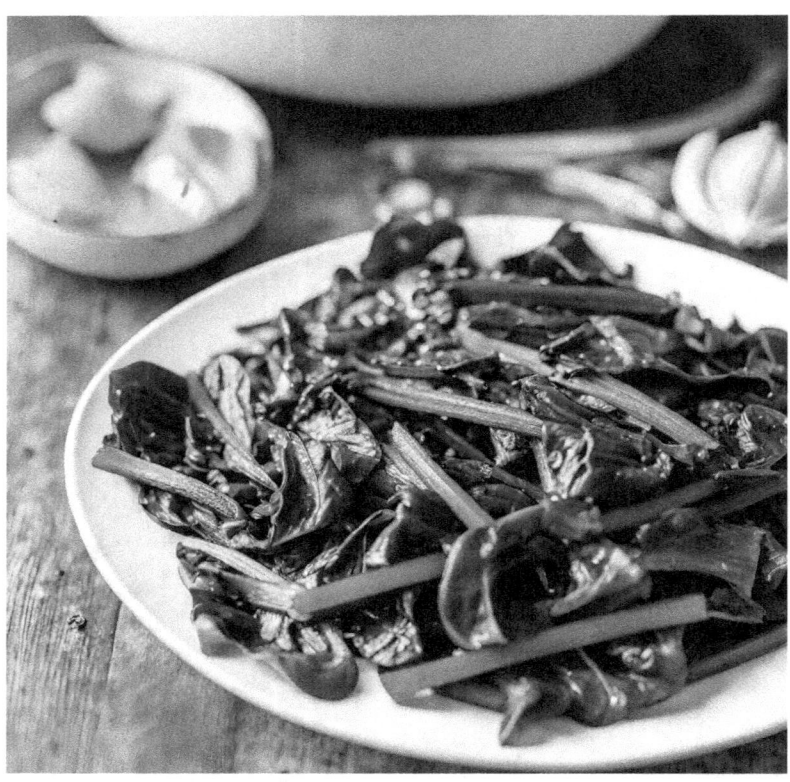

18. Grilled Zucchini Rolls with Herbed Cheese

Ingredients:
- 2 large zucchinis, sliced lengthwise into thin strips
- 1 cup herbed goat cheese or ricotta
- 2 tablespoons olive oil
- Fresh herbs (such as basil or thyme), for garnish

Instructions:
1. Preheat the grill to medium-high heat.
2. Brush zucchini strips with olive oil and grill until tender and grill marks appear, about 2-3 minutes per side.
3. Allow zucchini to cool slightly.
4. Spread each strip with a thin layer of herbed cheese.
5. Roll up strips and secure with a toothpick.
6. Garnish with fresh herbs before serving.

Nutrition Info (per serving, serves 4):
- Calories: 200
- Protein: 8 g
- Carbohydrates: 6 g
- Fat: 16 g
- Fiber: 1 g

Cooking Time: 20 minutes

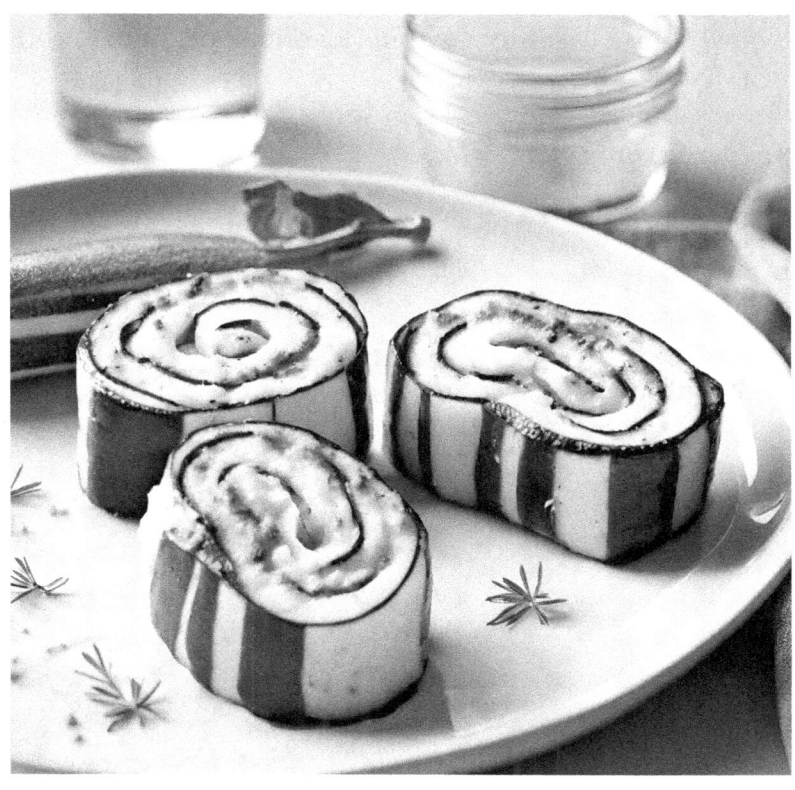

Beef & Pork Recipes

1. Beef Stir-Fry
Ingredients:
- 1 pound lean beef strips
- 2 tablespoons olive oil
- 1 bell pepper, sliced
- 1 onion, sliced
- 1 cup broccoli florets
- 2 cloves garlic, minced
- 1/4 cup soy sauce (low sodium)
- 1 tablespoon sesame oil
- 1 teaspoon honey
- 1 teaspoon grated ginger

Instructions:
1. Heat olive oil in a large skillet or wok over medium-high heat.
2. Add beef strips and stir-fry until browned and nearly cooked through, about 3-4 minutes.
3. Add garlic, bell pepper, onion, and broccoli. Continue to stir-fry until vegetables are tender-crisp, about 5 minutes.
4. In a small bowl, whisk together soy sauce, sesame oil, honey, and ginger. Pour over the stir-fry and toss to coat.
5. Cook for an additional 2 minutes, then serve hot.

Nutrition Info (per serving, serves 4):
- Calories: 300
- Protein: 26 g
- Carbohydrates: 10 g
- Fat: 18 g
- Fiber: 2 g

Cooking Time: 20 minutes

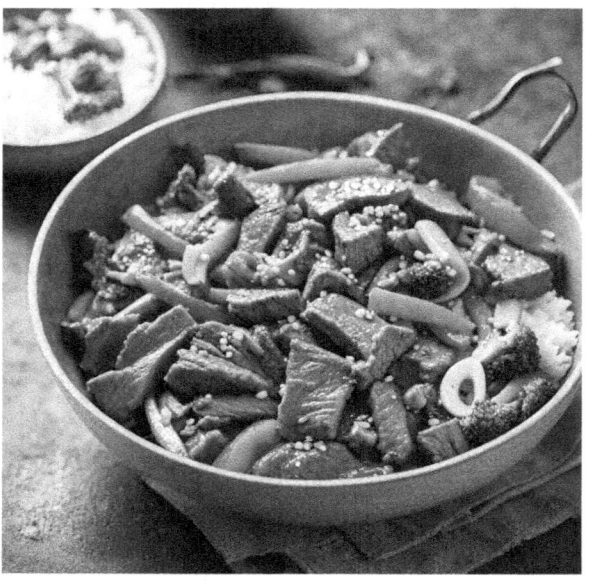

2. Pork Tenderloin

Ingredients:
- 1 pork tenderloin (about 1 pound)
- 2 tablespoons olive oil
- 1 teaspoon thyme
- 1 teaspoon rosemary
- 1 garlic clove, minced
- 1/2 cup chicken broth

Instructions:
1. Preheat oven to 375°F (190°C).
2. Rub pork tenderloin with olive oil, thyme, rosemary, and minced garlic.
3. Place in a roasting pan and pour chicken broth around it.
4. Roast in the preheated oven for 25-30 minutes, or until a meat thermometer inserted into the thickest part reads 145°F (63°C).
5. Let rest for 5 minutes before slicing and serving.

Nutrition Info (per serving, serves 4):
- Calories: 220
- Protein: 24 g
- Carbohydrates: 1 g
- Fat: 13 g
- Fiber: 0 g

Cooking Time: 35 minutes

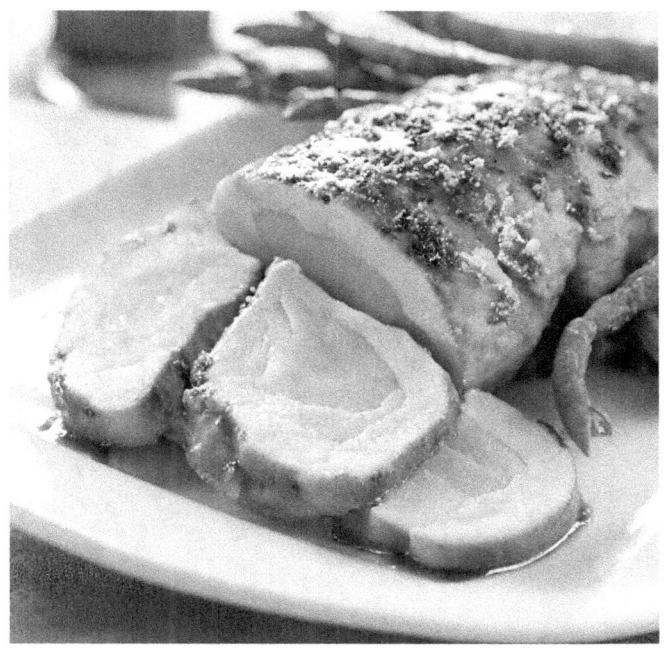

3. Beef and Vegetable Soup

Ingredients:
- 1 pound lean beef, cubed
- 2 tablespoons olive oil
- 1 onion, chopped
- 2 carrots, sliced
- 2 celery stalks, sliced
- 1 potato, cubed
- 4 cups beef broth
- 1 cup diced tomatoes
- 1 teaspoon dried basil
- 1 cup green beans, chopped

Instructions:
1. Heat olive oil in a large pot over medium heat.
2. Add beef and brown on all sides.
3. Add onion, carrots, and celery and sauté until vegetables are softened, about 5 minutes.
4. Add potatoes, beef broth, diced tomatoes, and basil. Bring to a boil.
5. Reduce heat to low and simmer for 1 hour.
6. Add green beans and cook for an additional 10 minutes.
7. Serve hot.

Nutrition Info (per serving, serves 6):
- Calories: 250
- Protein: 20 g
- Carbohydrates: 15 g
- Fat: 12 g
- Fiber: 3 g

Cooking Time: 1 hour 20 minutes

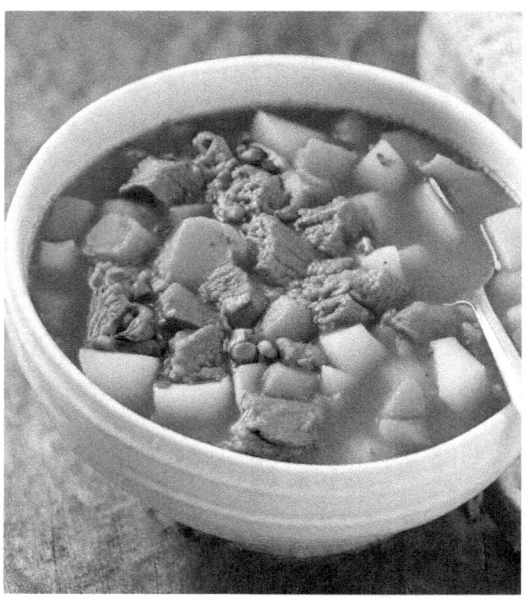

4. Beef Stroganoff

Ingredients:
- 1 pound lean beef strips
- 2 tablespoons olive oil
- 1 onion, chopped
- 2 cups mushrooms, sliced
- 1 cup beef broth
- 1 cup sour cream (low-fat)
- 1 tablespoon Dijon mustard
- 1 teaspoon paprika
- 1/4 cup parsley, chopped

Instructions:
1. Heat olive oil in a large skillet over medium-high heat.
2. Add beef and brown quickly on all sides. Remove from skillet and set aside.
3. In the same skillet, add onions and mushrooms. Cook until softened, about 5 minutes.
4. Return beef to the skillet and add beef broth. Simmer for 10 minutes.
5. Reduce heat to low and stir in sour cream, Dijon mustard, and paprika. Cook gently until heated through (do not boil).
6. Sprinkle with parsley before serving.

Nutrition Info (per serving, serves 4):
- Calories: 320
- Protein: 27 g
- Carbohydrates: 10 g
- Fat: 20 g
- Fiber: 2 g

Cooking Time: 30 minutes

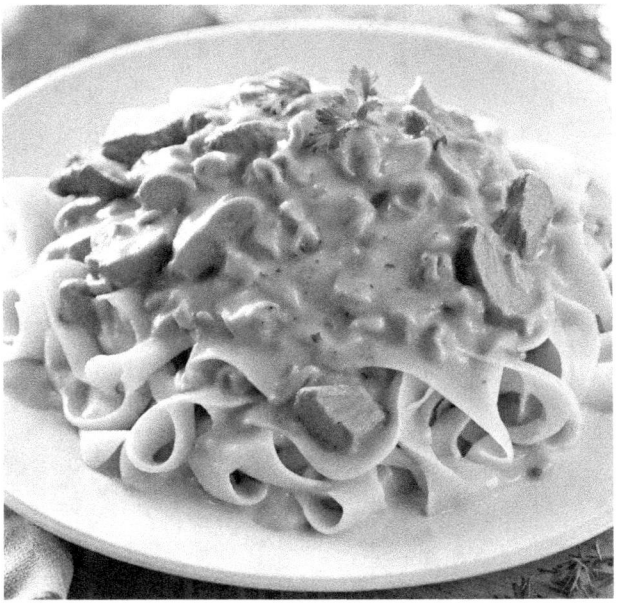

5. Pork Chops with Apples and Onions

Ingredients:
- 4 pork chops
- 2 tablespoons olive oil
- 2 apples, sliced
- 1 onion, sliced
- 1/2 cup apple cider
- 1 teaspoon thyme

Instructions:
1. Heat olive oil in a large skillet over medium-high heat.
2. Add pork chops and sear until golden, about 4 minutes per side.
3. Remove pork chops and add apples and onions to the skillet.
4. Sauté until softened, about 5 minutes.
5. Return pork chops to the skillet, add apple cider and thyme.
6. Cover and simmer for 10-15 minutes, or until pork chops are cooked through.
7. Serve pork chops topped with apples and onions.

Nutrition Info (per serving, serves 4):
- Calories: 350
- Protein: 29 g
- Carbohydrates: 15 g
- Fat: 19 g
- Fiber: 2 g

Cooking Time: 30 minutes

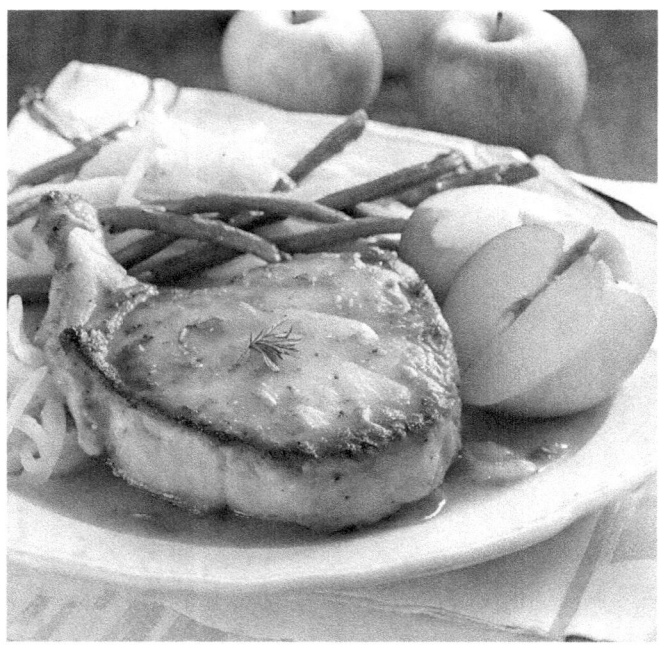

6. Italian Meatballs

Ingredients:
- 1 pound ground beef (lean)
- 1/2 cup breadcrumbs (gluten-free if necessary)
- 1/4 cup grated Parmesan cheese
- 1 egg
- 2 cloves garlic, minced
- 1 tablespoon dried basil
- 1 tablespoon dried oregano
- 1 cup marinara sauce (low sodium)

Instructions:
1. Preheat oven to 375°F (190°C).
2. In a large bowl, mix ground beef, breadcrumbs, Parmesan, egg, garlic, basil, and oregano until well combined.
3. Form mixture into 1-inch meatballs and place on a baking sheet lined with parchment paper.
4. Bake for 20-25 minutes, until meatballs are browned and cooked through.
5. Heat marinara sauce in a saucepan and add cooked meatballs. Simmer for 10 minutes.
6. Serve hot, garnished with extra Parmesan if desired.

Nutrition Info (per serving, serves 4):
- Calories: 320
- Protein: 26 g
- Carbohydrates: 15 g
- Fat: 17 g
- Fiber: 2 g

Cooking Time: 45 minutes

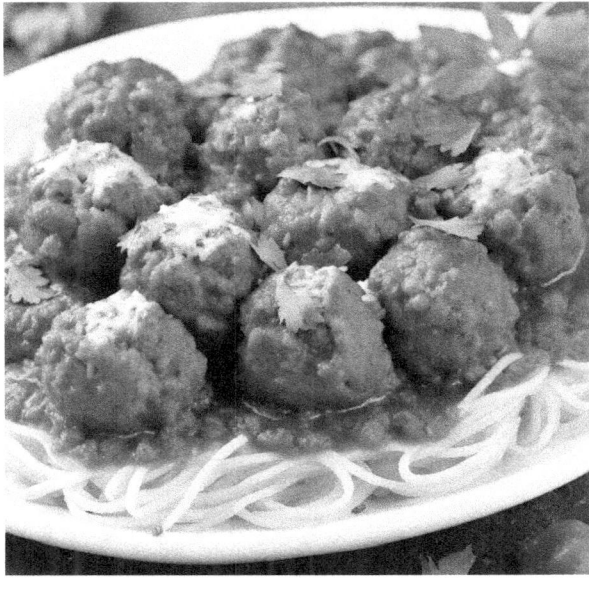

7. Beef Kabobs

Ingredients:
- 1 pound beef sirloin, cut into 1-inch cubes
- 2 bell peppers, cut into 1-inch pieces
- 1 onion, cut into wedges
- 2 zucchinis, sliced
- Marinade:
    - 1/4 cup olive oil
    - 2 tablespoons soy sauce (low sodium)
    - 1 tablespoon honey
    - 1 tablespoon garlic, minced
    - 1 teaspoon dried thyme

Instructions:
1. In a bowl, whisk together olive oil, soy sauce, honey, garlic, and thyme to make the marinade.
2. Add beef cubes to the marinade and let sit for at least 30 minutes in the refrigerator.
3. Preheat the grill to medium-high heat.
4. Thread marinated beef, bell peppers, onions, and zucchinis onto skewers.
5. Grill kabobs, turning occasionally, until beef is cooked to desired doneness and vegetables are tender, about 10-15 minutes.
6. Serve hot.

Nutrition Info (per serving, serves 4):
- Calories: 350
- Protein: 25 g
- Carbohydrates: 15 g
- Fat: 20 g
- Fiber: 3 g

Cooking Time: 55 minutes (including marinating time)

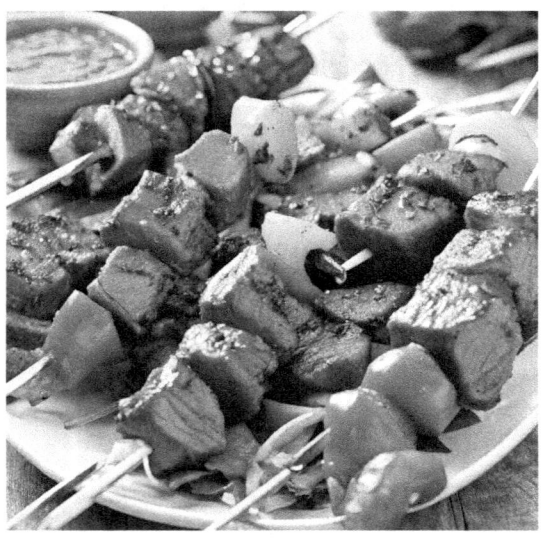

8. Pork and Sweet Potato Stew

Ingredients:
- 1 pound pork shoulder, cubed
- 2 sweet potatoes, peeled and cubed
- 1 onion, chopped
- 2 carrots, sliced
- 4 cups chicken broth
- 2 tablespoons olive oil
- 1 teaspoon paprika
- 1 teaspoon dried thyme

Instructions:
1. Heat olive oil in a large pot over medium heat.
2. Add pork cubes and brown on all sides.
3. Add onions and carrots, cooking until softened.
4. Add sweet potatoes, chicken broth, paprika, and thyme.
5. Bring to a boil, then reduce heat and simmer for about 1 hour until pork is tender.
6. Serve hot.

Nutrition Info (per serving, serves 4):
- Calories: 400
- Protein: 25 g
- Carbohydrates: 30 g
- Fat: 20 g
- Fiber: 5 g

Cooking Time: 1 hour 20 minutes

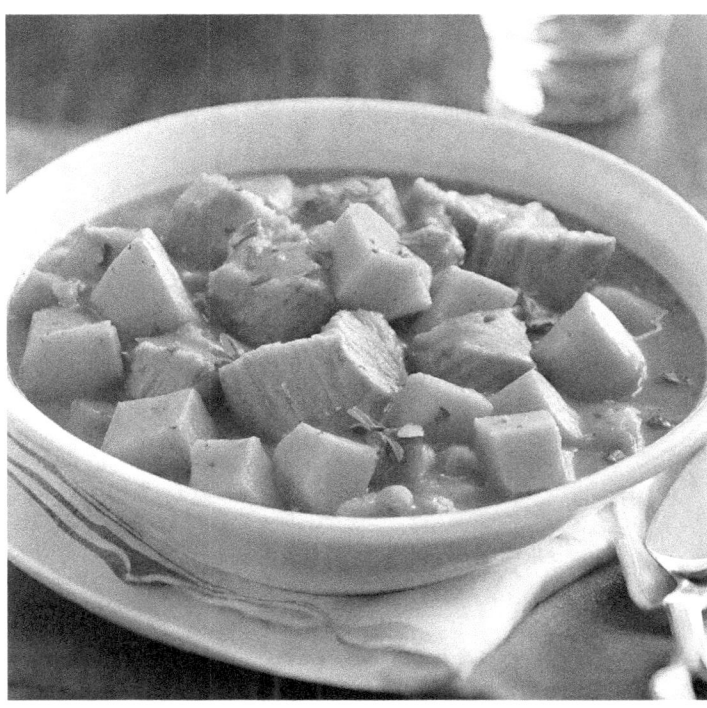

9. Pork Loin Roast

Ingredients:
- 1 pork loin roast (about 3 pounds)
- 2 tablespoons olive oil
- 1 tablespoon garlic, minced
- 2 teaspoons dried rosemary
- 1/2 cup white wine
- 1 cup chicken broth

Instructions:
1. Preheat oven to 350°F (175°C).
2. Rub pork loin with olive oil, garlic, and rosemary.
3. Place in a roasting pan and roast for about 1 hour.
4. Deglaze the pan with white wine, add chicken broth, and continue cooking for another 30 minutes or until the internal temperature reaches 145°F (63°C).
5. Let rest before slicing.

Nutrition Info (per serving, serves 6):
- Calories: 300
- Protein: 35 g
- Carbohydrates: 2 g
- Fat: 16 g
- Fiber: 0 g

Cooking Time: 1 hour 30 minutes

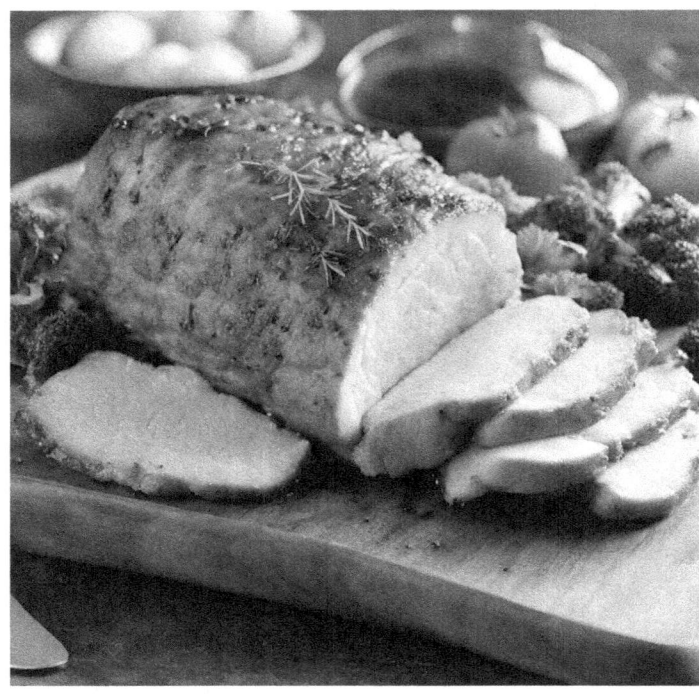

10. Balsamic Glazed Beef

Ingredients:
- 1 pound beef sirloin, sliced into strips
- 1/4 cup balsamic vinegar
- 2 tablespoons honey
- 1 tablespoon olive oil
- 1 onion, sliced
- 1 red bell pepper, sliced

Instructions:
1. Heat olive oil in a skillet over medium-high heat.
2. Add beef and cook until browned.
3. Remove beef and add onion and bell pepper to the skillet. Sauté until soft.
4. Return beef to skillet and add balsamic vinegar and honey. Cook until sauce thickens.
5. Serve hot.

Nutrition Info (per serving, serves 4):
- Calories: 250
- Protein: 25 g
- Carbohydrates: 15 g
- Fat: 10 g
- Fiber: 1 g

Cooking Time: 30 minutes

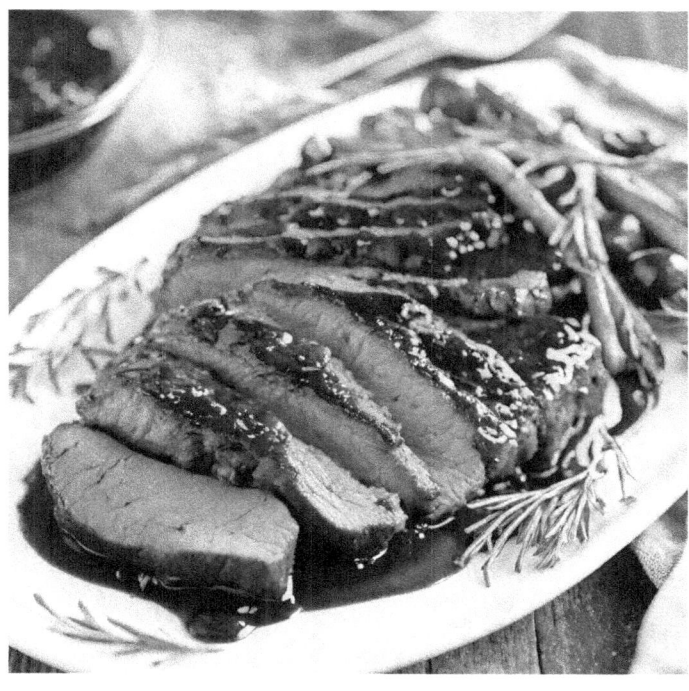

11. Spiced Pork Ribs

Ingredients:
- 2 pounds pork ribs
- 1/4 cup apple cider vinegar
- 2 tablespoons honey
- 1 tablespoon smoked paprika
- 1 teaspoon cumin
- 1 teaspoon dried oregano
- 2 tablespoons olive oil

Instructions:
1. Preheat oven to 300°F (150°C).
2. Mix together vinegar, honey, paprika, cumin, and oregano.
3. Rub ribs with olive oil and spice mixture.
4. Wrap ribs in foil and bake for 3 hours until tender.
5. Unwrap and broil for 5 minutes to crisp.

Nutrition Info (per serving, serves 4):
- Calories: 500
- Protein: 30 g
- Carbohydrates: 15 g
- Fat: 35 g
- Fiber: 1 g

Cooking Time: 3 hours 10 minutes

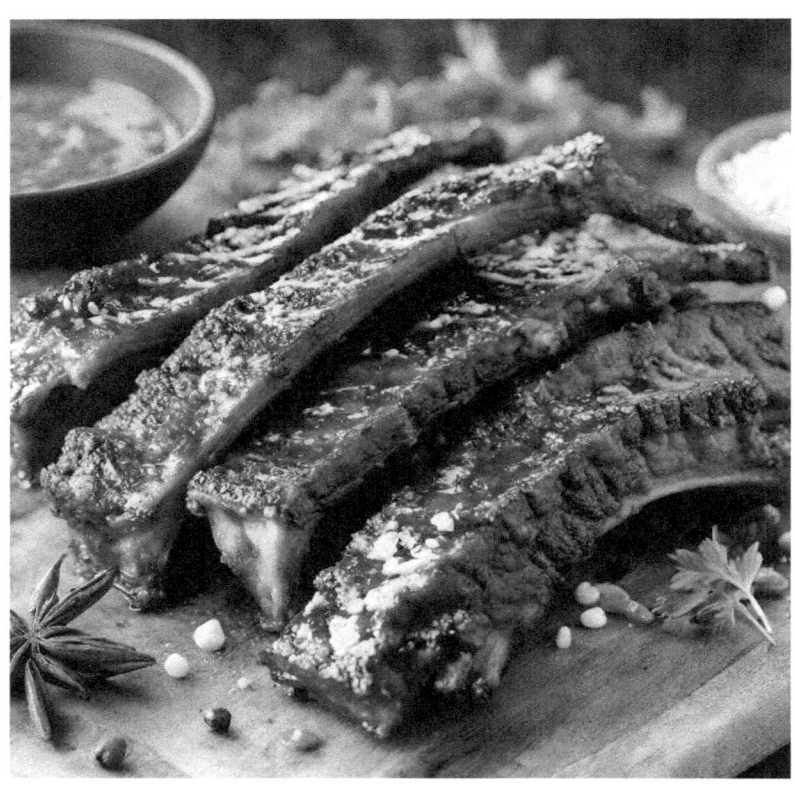

12. Beef Bourguignon

Ingredients:
- 1.5 pounds beef chuck, cut into cubes
- 3 tablespoons olive oil
- 1 onion, chopped
- 2 carrots, sliced
- 2 cloves garlic, minced
- 1/2 bottle dry red wine (about 375 ml)
- 2 cups beef broth
- 1 tablespoon tomato paste
- 1 teaspoon dried thyme
- 1 bay leaf
- 1 cup pearl onions, peeled
- 1 cup mushrooms, quartered

Instructions:
1. Heat 2 tablespoons of olive oil in a large pot over medium-high heat. Brown the beef cubes on all sides and set aside.
2. In the same pot, add the remaining olive oil and cook the onion, carrots, and garlic until softened.
3. Return the beef to the pot. Stir in the red wine, beef broth, tomato paste, thyme, and bay leaf. Bring to a simmer.
4. Cover and cook on low heat for 1.5 hours.
5. Add pearl onions and mushrooms, and cook for another 30 minutes until the vegetables are tender and the beef is very tender.
6. Remove the bay leaf and serve.

Nutrition Info (per serving, serves 6):
- Calories: 380
- Protein: 25 g
- Carbohydrates: 15 g
- Fat: 20 g
- Fiber: 3 g

Cooking Time: 2 hours 10 minutes

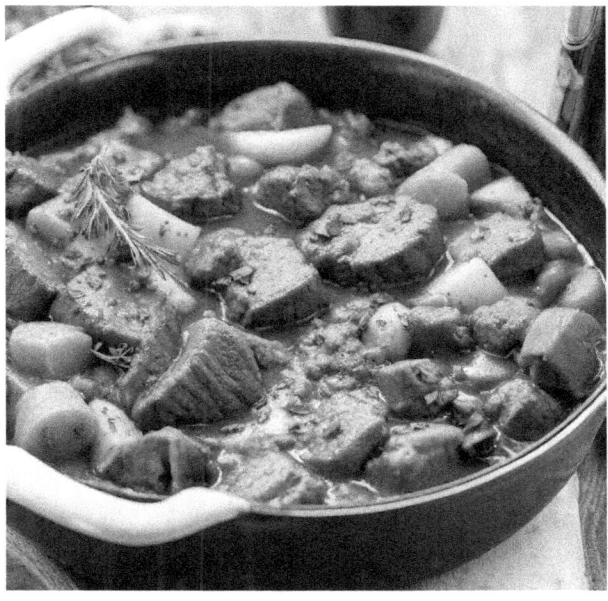

13. Pork Scallopini

Ingredients:
- 1 pound pork tenderloin, thinly sliced
- 1/4 cup flour (gluten-free if needed)
- 2 tablespoons olive oil
- 1/2 cup chicken broth
- 1 lemon, juiced
- 1 tablespoon capers
- 1/4 cup fresh parsley, chopped

Instructions:
1. Dredge pork slices in flour, shaking off the excess.
2. Heat olive oil in a skillet over medium-high heat. Add pork and cook until golden and cooked through, about 2 minutes per side.
3. Remove pork from skillet and keep warm.
4. Add chicken broth, lemon juice, and capers to the skillet. Bring to a boil and cook until slightly thickened.
5. Return pork to the skillet and coat with the sauce.
6. Garnish with fresh parsley before serving.

Nutrition Info (per serving, serves 4):
- Calories: 280
- Protein: 26 g
- Carbohydrates: 9 g
- Fat: 15 g
- Fiber: 1 g

Cooking Time: 20 minutes

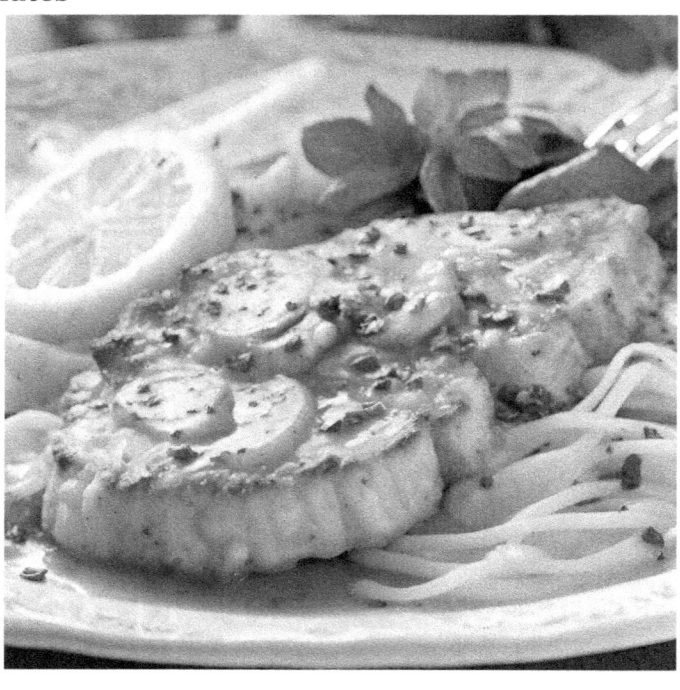

14. Beef Chili

Ingredients:
- 1 pound lean ground beef
- 1 onion, chopped
- 2 cloves garlic, minced
- 1 can (15 oz) diced tomatoes
- 1 can (15 oz) kidney beans, drained and rinsed
- 2 tablespoons chili powder
- 1 teaspoon cumin
- 1 cup beef broth

Instructions:
1. In a large pot, cook ground beef over medium heat until browned. Drain excess fat.
2. Add onion and garlic, and cook until soft.
3. Stir in diced tomatoes, kidney beans, chili powder, cumin, and beef broth. Bring to a boil.
4. Reduce heat and simmer for 45 minutes, stirring occasionally.
5. Serve hot.

Nutrition Info (per serving, serves 4):
- Calories: 350
- Protein: 30 g
- Carbohydrates: 25 g
- Fat: 15 g
- Fiber: 7 g

Cooking Time: 1 hour

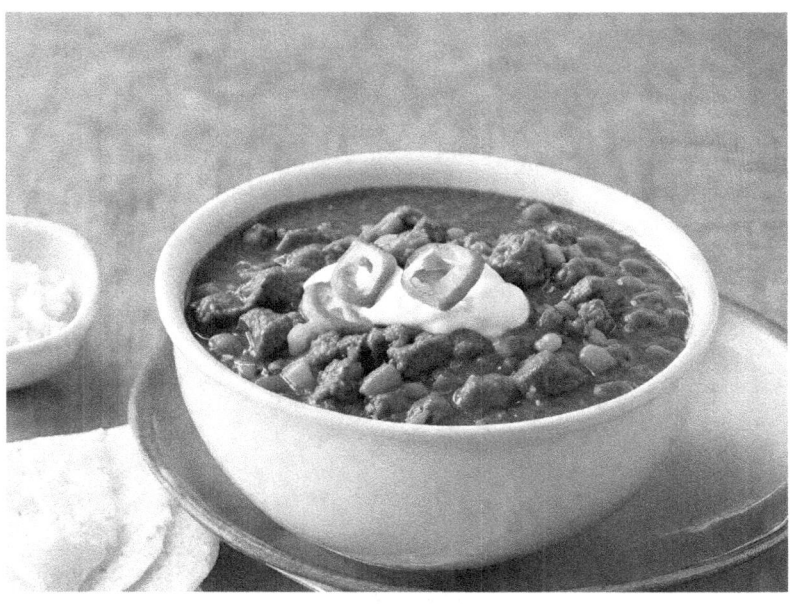

15. Ginger Pork Stir-Fry

Ingredients:
- 1 pound pork loin, thinly sliced
- 2 tablespoons olive oil
- 1 bell pepper, sliced
- 1 onion, sliced
- 2 tablespoons grated ginger
- 1/4 cup soy sauce (low sodium)
- 1 tablespoon honey
- 1/2 cup sliced green onions

Instructions:
1. Heat olive oil in a large skillet over medium-high heat. Add pork and stir-fry until browned.
2. Add bell pepper, onion, and ginger. Continue to stir-fry until vegetables are tender.
3. Stir in soy sauce and honey, cooking for an additional 2 minutes until the sauce is slightly thickened.
4. Garnish with green onions and serve.

Nutrition Info (per serving, serves 4):
- Calories: 280
- Protein: 25 g
- Carbohydrates: 15 g
- Fat: 14 g
- Fiber: 2 g

Cooking Time: 20 minutes

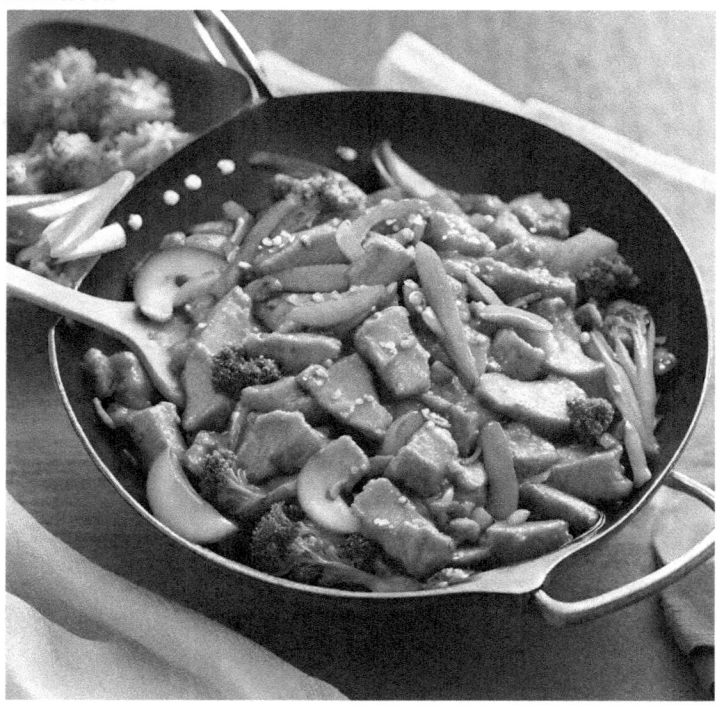

16. Beef Brisket

Ingredients:
- 3 pounds beef brisket
- 2 tablespoons olive oil
- 1 onion, sliced
- 3 cloves garlic, minced
- 1 cup beef broth
- 1/2 cup apple cider vinegar
- 1 tablespoon honey
- 1 tablespoon smoked paprika

Instructions:
1. Preheat oven to 300°F (150°C).
2. Heat olive oil in a large skillet over medium-high heat. Sear the brisket on both sides until browned.
3. Transfer brisket to a roasting pan. In the same skillet, sauté onion and garlic until soft.
4. Add beef broth, apple cider vinegar, honey, and smoked paprika to the skillet, stirring to combine. Bring to a simmer.
5. Pour the mixture over the brisket. Cover the roasting pan with foil.
6. Roast in the preheated oven for about 3 hours, or until the brisket is tender.
7. Slice and serve with the cooking juices.

Nutrition Info (per serving, serves 6):
- Calories: 480
- Protein: 60 g
- Carbohydrates: 10 g
- Fat: 22 g
- Fiber: 1 g

Cooking Time: 3 hours 15 minutes

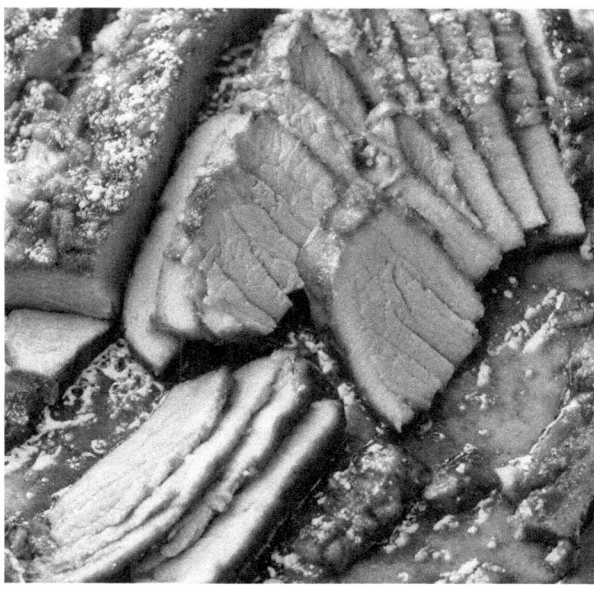

17. Pork Carnitas

Ingredients:
- 2 pounds pork shoulder, cut into chunks
- 1 onion, chopped
- 3 cloves garlic, minced
- 1 orange, juiced
- 1 lime, juiced
- 1 teaspoon cumin
- 1 teaspoon dried oregano
- 2 cups chicken broth

Instructions:
1. Place pork shoulder, onion, garlic, orange juice, lime juice, cumin, and oregano in a slow cooker.
2. Pour chicken broth over the ingredients.
3. Cook on low for 8 hours until the pork is tender and shreds easily.
4. Shred the pork using two forks and serve with tortillas or over rice.

Nutrition Info (per serving, serves 6):
- Calories: 350
- Protein: 30 g
- Carbohydrates: 6 g
- Fat: 22 g
- Fiber: 1 g

Cooking Time: 8 hours

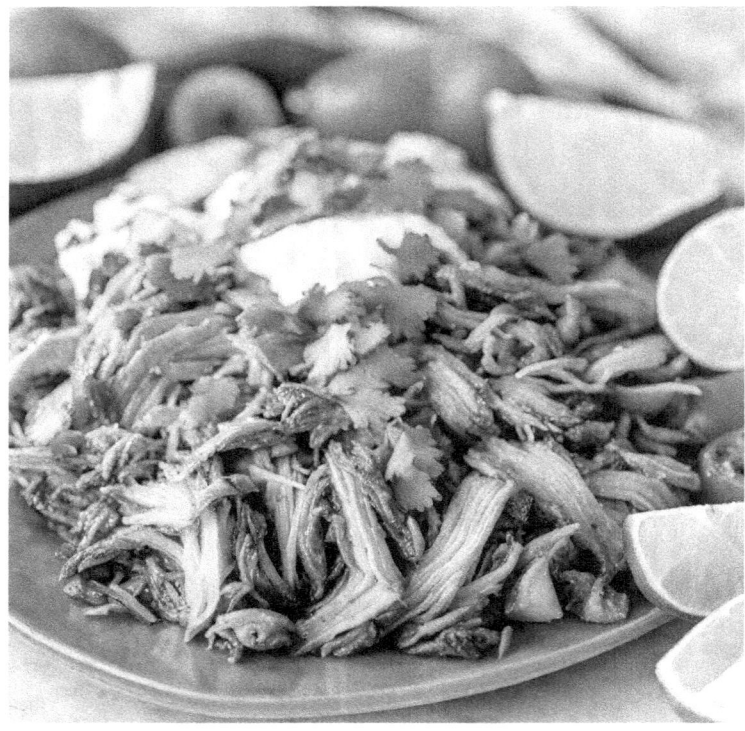

18. Beef Tenderloin with Herb Crust

Ingredients:
- 2 pounds beef tenderloin
- 2 tablespoons Dijon mustard
- 1 cup fresh herbs (parsley, thyme, rosemary), finely chopped
- 2 tablespoons olive oil
- 1/4 cup breadcrumbs (gluten-free if needed)

Instructions:
1. Preheat oven to 400°F (200°C).
2. Rub the beef tenderloin with Dijon mustard.
3. In a bowl, mix together the chopped herbs, olive oil, and breadcrumbs.
4. Coat the mustard-rubbed tenderloin with the herb and breadcrumb mixture.
5. Roast in the preheated oven for about 30 minutes, or until a meat thermometer inserted into the center reads 135°F (57°C) for medium-rare.
6. Let rest for 10 minutes before slicing.

Nutrition Info (per serving, serves 6):
- Calories: 450
- Protein: 45 g
- Carbohydrates: 4 g
- Fat: 28 g
- Fiber: 1 g

Cooking Time: 40 minutes

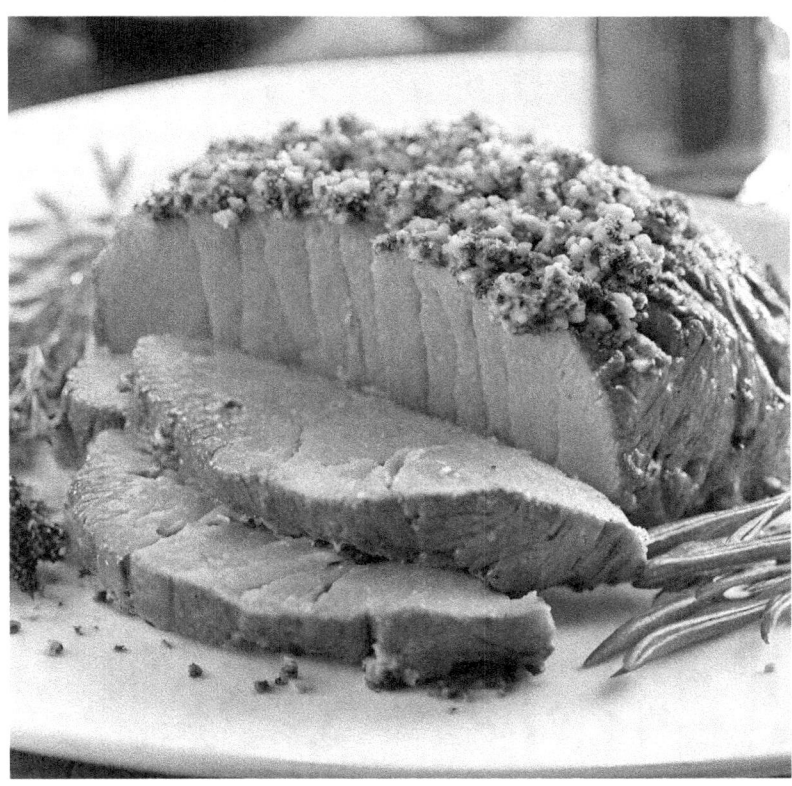

19. Pork Vegetable Soup

Ingredients:
- 1 pound pork loin, cubed
- 2 carrots, chopped
- 2 potatoes, chopped
- 1 onion, chopped
- 4 cups chicken broth
- 1 cup diced tomatoes
- 1 teaspoon thyme
- 2 tablespoons olive oil

Instructions:
1. Heat olive oil in a large pot over medium heat.
2. Add pork loin and brown on all sides.
3. Add onions, carrots, and potatoes, sautéing until slightly softened.
4. Pour in chicken broth and diced tomatoes. Bring to a boil.
5. Reduce heat and simmer for 30 minutes, or until vegetables are tender and pork is cooked through.
6. Stir in thyme and cook for an additional 5 minutes.
7. Serve hot.

Nutrition Info (per serving, serves 6):
- Calories: 250
- Protein: 20 g
- Carbohydrates: 20 g
- Fat: 10 g
- Fiber: 3 g

Cooking Time: 45 minutes

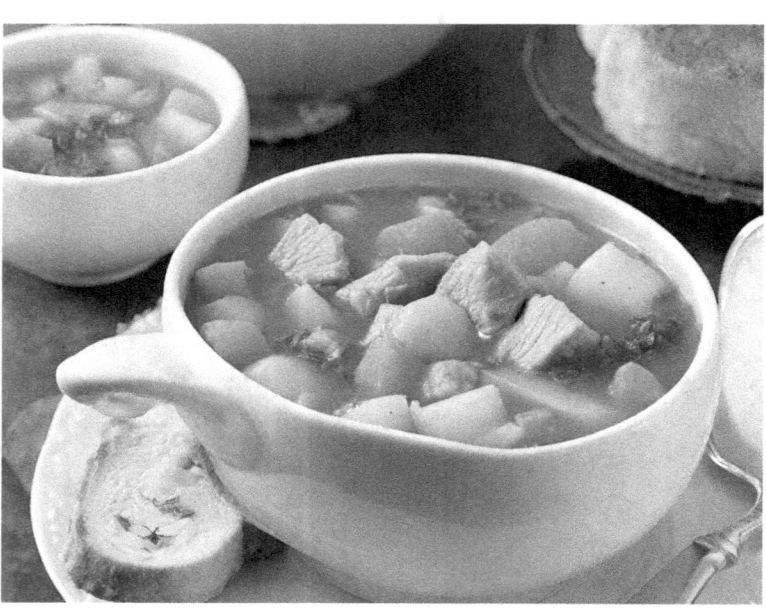

20. Beef Goulash

Ingredients:
- 2 pounds beef stew meat, cubed
- 2 tablespoons olive oil
- 1 large onion, chopped
- 2 cloves garlic, minced
- 1 bell pepper, chopped
- 2 tablespoons paprika
- 1 can (14 oz) diced tomatoes
- 2 cups beef broth
- 1 cup sour cream (low-fat)
- 1 tablespoon fresh parsley, chopped

Instructions:
1. Heat olive oil in a large pot over medium-high heat.
2. Brown the beef cubes on all sides and set aside.
3. In the same pot, sauté onion, garlic, and bell pepper until soft.
4. Add paprika and stir for about 1 minute until fragrant.
5. Return the beef to the pot, add diced tomatoes and beef broth. Bring to a boil, then reduce heat and simmer for about 1.5 hours, or until the beef is tender.
6. Stir in sour cream and heat through (do not boil).
7. Garnish with fresh parsley before serving.

Nutrition Info (per serving, serves 6):
- Calories: 400
- Protein: 35 g
- Carbohydrates: 10 g
- Fat: 25 g
- Fiber: 2 g

Cooking Time: 1 hour 50 minutes

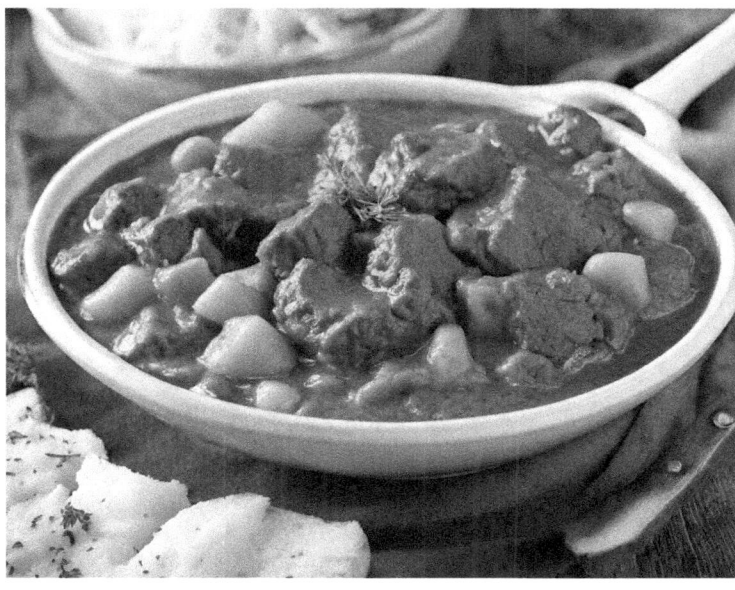

21. Beef Ragout

Ingredients:
- 1.5 pounds beef chuck, cut into cubes
- 1 onion, diced
- 2 carrots, sliced
- 2 celery stalks, sliced
- 3 cloves garlic, minced
- 1 cup red wine
- 2 cups beef broth
- 1 can (14 oz) crushed tomatoes
- 1 teaspoon thyme
- 2 tablespoons olive oil

Instructions:
1. Heat olive oil in a large pot over medium-high heat.
2. Brown the beef cubes on all sides and set aside.
3. In the same pot, sauté onion, carrots, celery, and garlic until softened.
4. Deglaze the pot with red wine, scraping up any browned bits.
5. Add beef broth, crushed tomatoes, thyme, and return the beef to the pot.
6. Simmer covered for 2 hours, or until the beef is tender.
7. Adjust seasoning and serve hot.

Nutrition Info (per serving, serves 6):
- Calories: 380
- Protein: 30 g
- Carbohydrates: 15 g
- Fat: 20 g
- Fiber: 3 g

Cooking Time: 2 hours 30 minutes

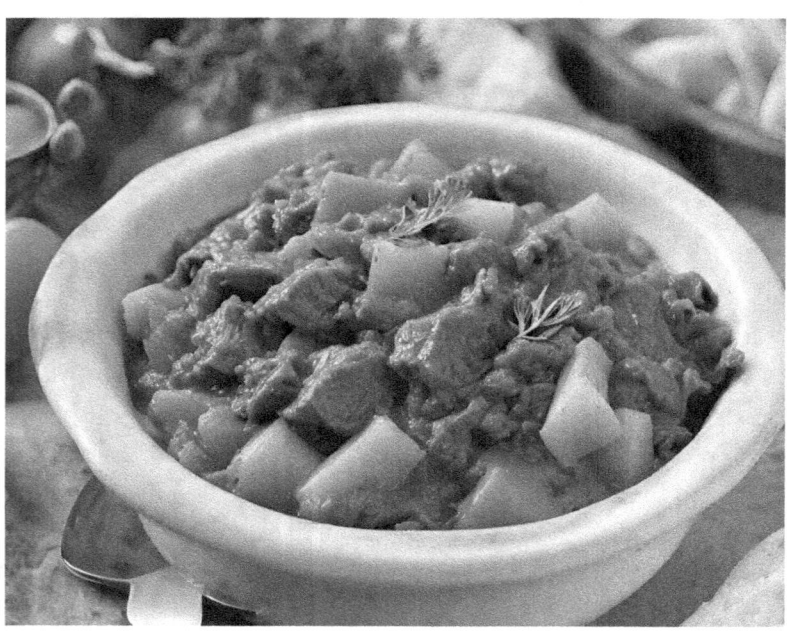

22. Herb-Crusted Pork Medallions

Ingredients:
- 1 pound pork tenderloin, sliced into 1-inch thick medallions
- 1/4 cup breadcrumbs (gluten-free if needed)
- 1/4 cup fresh herbs (parsley, thyme, rosemary), finely chopped
- 1 egg, beaten
- 2 tablespoons olive oil

Instructions:
1. Dip each pork medallion into the beaten egg, then coat with a mixture of breadcrumbs and chopped herbs.
2. Heat olive oil in a skillet over medium-high heat.
3. Cook the pork medallions for about 3-4 minutes on each side or until golden brown and cooked through.
4. Serve hot.

Nutrition Info (per serving, serves 4):
- Calories: 250
- Protein: 25 g
- Carbohydrates: 8 g
- Fat: 13 g
- Fiber: 1 g

Cooking Time: 20 minutes

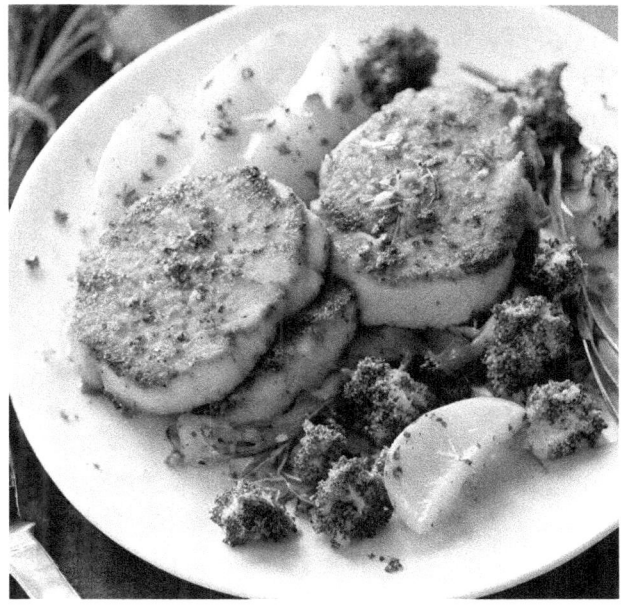

23. Beef Fajitas

Ingredients:
- 1 pound beef flank steak, thinly sliced
- 2 bell peppers, sliced
- 1 onion, sliced
- 2 tablespoons olive oil
- 1 teaspoon cumin
- 1 teaspoon chili powder
- 1/4 cup lime juice
- 4-6 small flour tortillas (gluten-free if needed)

Instructions:
1. In a large bowl, combine olive oil, cumin, chili powder, and lime juice. Add the beef, bell peppers, and onion, tossing to coat.
2. Heat a large skillet or grill pan over high heat.
3. Cook the beef and vegetables until the beef is browned and the vegetables are tender-crisp, about 5-6 minutes.
4. Serve with warm tortillas.

Nutrition Info (per serving, serves 4):
- Calories: 350
- Protein: 25 g
- Carbohydrates: 30 g
- Fat: 15 g
- Fiber: 3 g

Cooking Time: 25 minutes

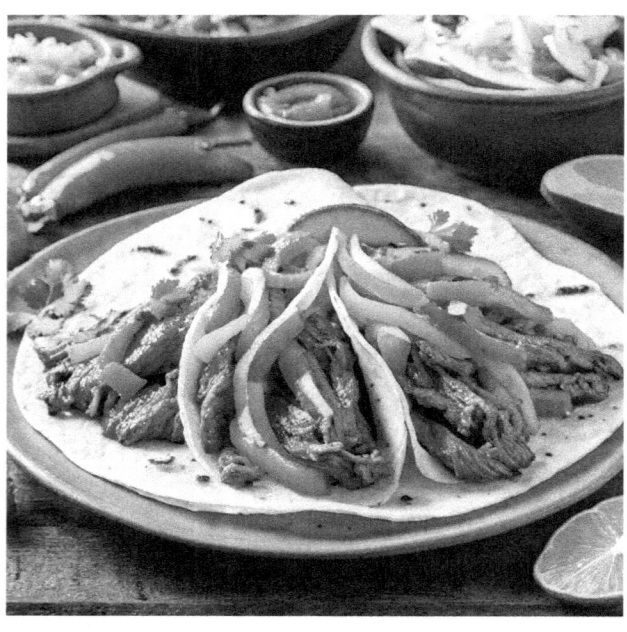

Fish & Seafood Recipes

1. Grilled Salmon with Lemon and Dill
Ingredients:
- 4 salmon fillets (6 ounces each)
- 2 tablespoons olive oil
- 1 lemon, juiced and zest grated
- 2 tablespoons fresh dill, chopped
- Lemon slices for garnish

Instructions:
1. Preheat the grill to medium heat.
2. In a small bowl, mix together olive oil, lemon juice, lemon zest, and dill.
3. Brush the salmon fillets with the lemon and dill mixture.
4. Place salmon on the grill, skin side down, and cook for 6-8 minutes on each side or until the fish flakes easily with a fork.
5. Serve garnished with lemon slices.

Nutrition Info (per serving, serves 4):
- Calories: 280
- Protein: 23 g
- Carbohydrates: 1 g
- Fat: 20 g
- Fiber: 0 g

Cooking Time: 16 minutes

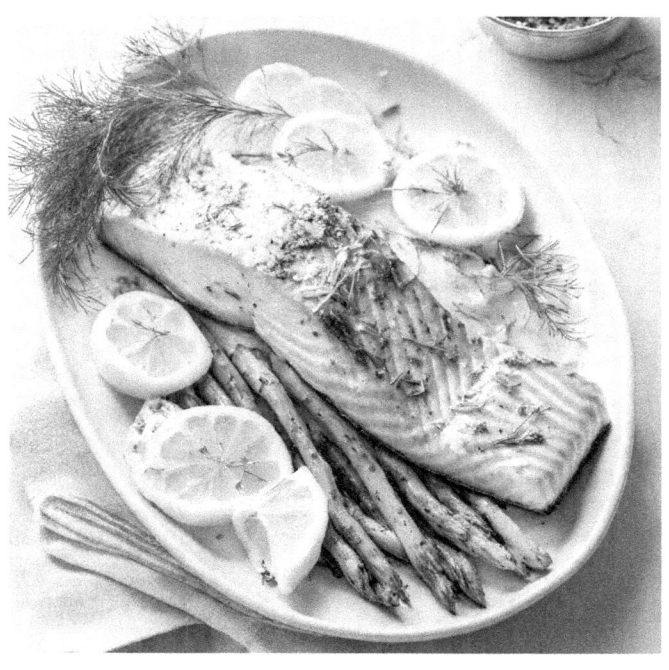

2. Shrimp Stir-Fry with Mixed Vegetables

Ingredients:
- 1 pound shrimp, peeled and deveined
- 2 cups mixed vegetables (carrots, bell peppers, broccoli)
- 2 tablespoons olive oil
- 1 tablespoon soy sauce (low sodium)
- 1 tablespoon ginger, minced
- 1 garlic clove, minced

Instructions:
1. Heat olive oil in a large skillet over medium-high heat.
2. Add garlic and ginger, sauté for 30 seconds.
3. Add shrimp and stir-fry until they turn pink, about 2-3 minutes.
4. Add mixed vegetables and soy sauce, continue to stir-fry until vegetables are tender-crisp, about 5 minutes.
5. Serve hot.

Nutrition Info (per serving, serves 4):
- Calories: 220
- Protein: 24 g
- Carbohydrates: 8 g
- Fat: 10 g
- Fiber: 2 g

Cooking Time: 10 minutes

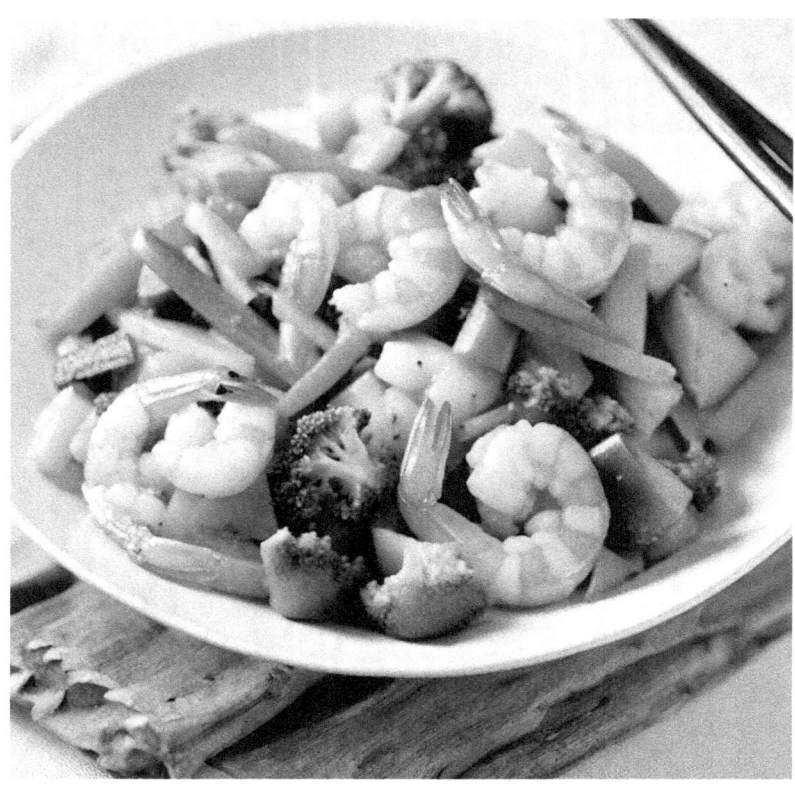

3. Baked Cod with Olive Tapenade

Ingredients:
- 4 cod fillets (6 ounces each)
- 1/2 cup olive tapenade
- 1 tablespoon olive oil
- Fresh parsley, chopped for garnish

Instructions:
1. Preheat oven to 400°F (200°C).
2. Place cod fillets in a baking dish and brush with olive oil.
3. Spread olive tapenade evenly over each fillet.
4. Bake for 12-15 minutes or until fish flakes easily with a fork.
5. Garnish with fresh parsley before serving.

Nutrition Info (per serving, serves 4):
- Calories: 220
- Protein: 25 g
- Carbohydrates: 2 g
- Fat: 12 g
- Fiber: 1 g

Cooking Time: 15 minutes

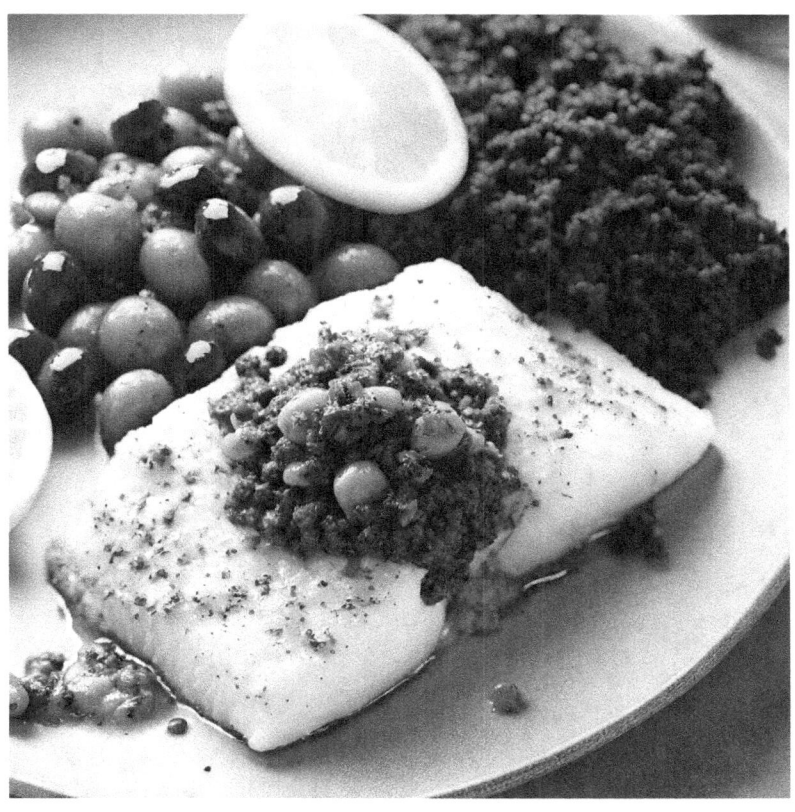

4. Pan-Seared Tuna Steaks

Ingredients:
- 4 tuna steaks (6 ounces each)
- 2 tablespoons olive oil
- 1 tablespoon sesame seeds
- 1 tablespoon soy sauce (low sodium)
- 1 teaspoon wasabi paste

Instructions:
1. Heat olive oil in a skillet over medium-high heat.
2. Rub each tuna steak with a little soy sauce and wasabi paste.
3. Coat the steaks with sesame seeds.
4. Sear the tuna for about 2 minutes on each side for medium-rare, or longer for well-done.
5. Serve immediately.

Nutrition Info (per serving, serves 4):
- Calories: 300
- Protein: 40 g
- Carbohydrates: 2 g
- Fat: 14 g
- Fiber: 1 g

Cooking Time: 10 minutes

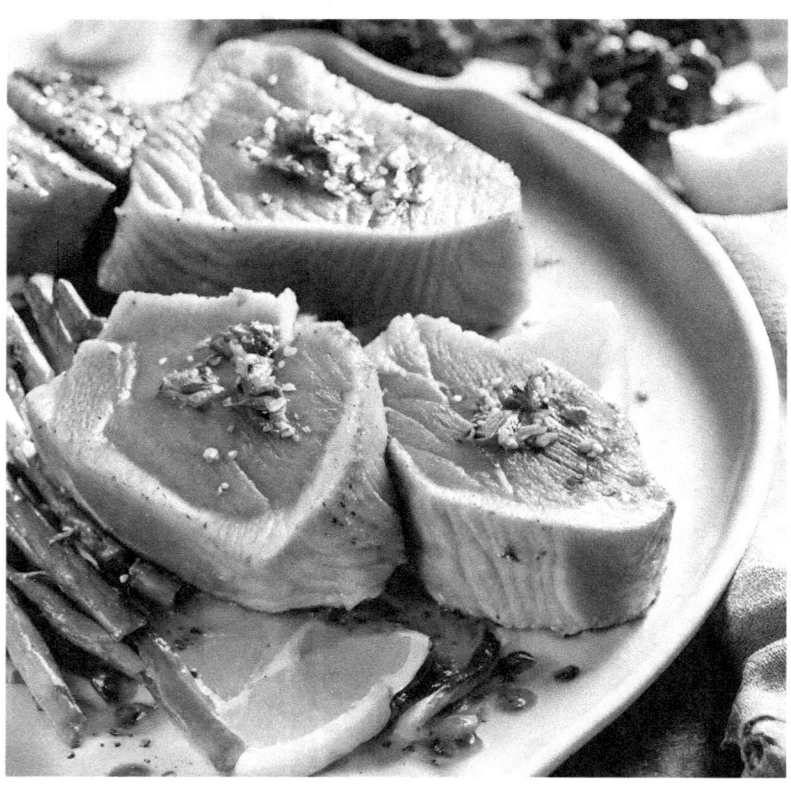

5. Seafood Paella with Brown Rice

Ingredients:
- 1 cup brown rice
- 2 cups fish stock
- 1/2 pound shrimp, peeled and deveined
- 1/2 pound mussels, cleaned
- 1/2 pound clams, cleaned
- 1/2 cup peas
- 1 onion, chopped
- 1 red bell pepper, chopped
- 2 tablespoons olive oil
- 1 teaspoon saffron threads
- 1 lemon, wedged for serving

Instructions:
1. Heat olive oil in a large skillet over medium heat. Add onion and bell pepper, sauté until soft.
2. Add rice and stir to coat with oil. Pour in fish stock and bring to a boil.
3. Reduce heat, add saffron, and simmer covered for 30 minutes.
4. Stir in shrimp, mussels, clams, and peas. Cover and cook until shellfish open and shrimp are cooked through, about 10 minutes.
5. Serve hot with lemon wedges.

Nutrition Info (per serving, serves 4):
- Calories: 400
- Protein: 30 g
- Carbohydrates: 42 g
- Fat: 12 g
- Fiber: 4 g

Cooking Time: 50 minutes

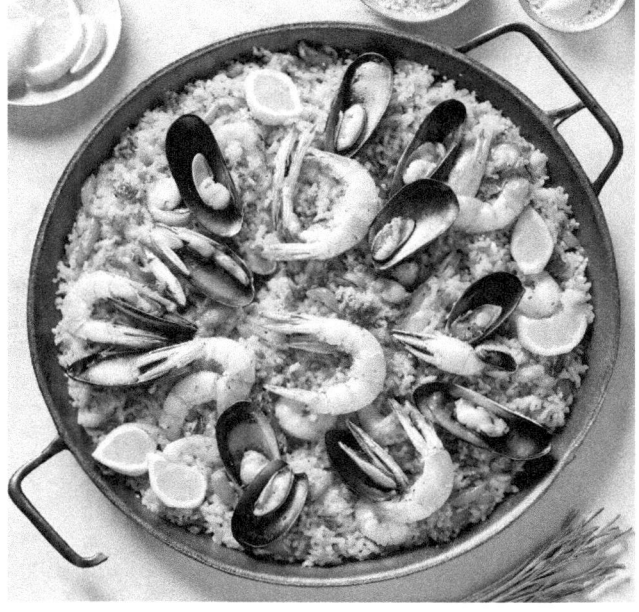

6. Mussels in Tomato Garlic Broth

Ingredients:
- 2 pounds mussels, cleaned and debearded
- 1 tablespoon olive oil
- 3 cloves garlic, minced
- 1 onion, chopped
- 1 can (14 oz) diced tomatoes
- 1/2 cup white wine
- 1/4 cup fresh parsley, chopped

Instructions:
1. Heat olive oil in a large pot over medium heat.
2. Add garlic and onion, and sauté until onion is translucent.
3. Pour in white wine and bring to a simmer.
4. Add diced tomatoes and bring to a boil.
5. Add mussels and cover the pot. Cook for 5-7 minutes until all mussels have opened (discard any that do not open).
6. Stir in fresh parsley just before serving.
7. Serve hot with crusty bread if desired.

Nutrition Info (per serving, serves 4):
- Calories: 240
- Protein: 18 g
- Carbohydrates: 10 g
- Fat: 10 g
- Fiber: 1 g

Cooking Time: 20 minutes

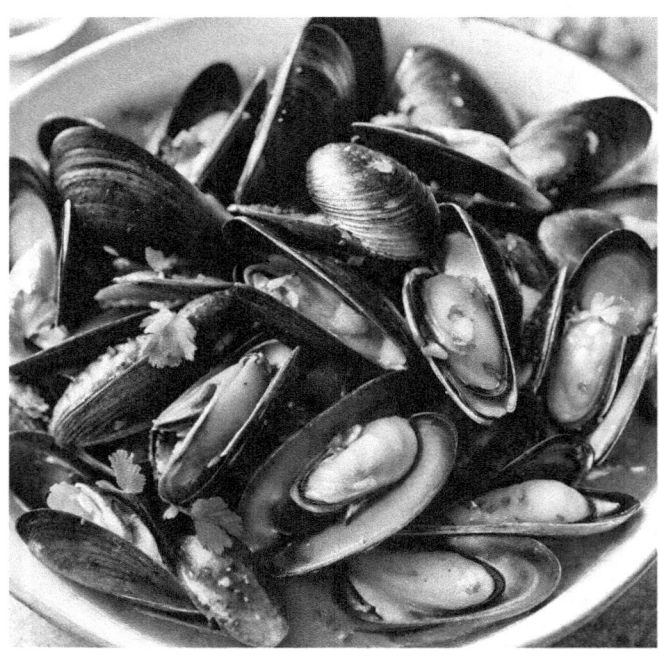

7. Crab Salad with Avocado and Cucumber

Ingredients:
- 1 pound crab meat, cooked and shredded
- 1 avocado, diced
- 1 cucumber, diced
- 1/4 cup mayonnaise (low-fat)
- 1 lemon, juiced
- 2 tablespoons fresh dill, chopped
- Lettuce leaves for serving

Instructions:
1. In a bowl, combine crab meat, avocado, cucumber, mayonnaise, lemon juice, and dill.
2. Gently mix until all ingredients are well coated.
3. Chill in the refrigerator for at least 30 minutes to blend flavors.
4. Serve on a bed of lettuce leaves.

Nutrition Info (per serving, serves 4):
- Calories: 280
- Protein: 22 g
- Carbohydrates: 8 g
- Fat: 18 g
- Fiber: 4 g

Cooking Time: 40 minutes (including chilling time)

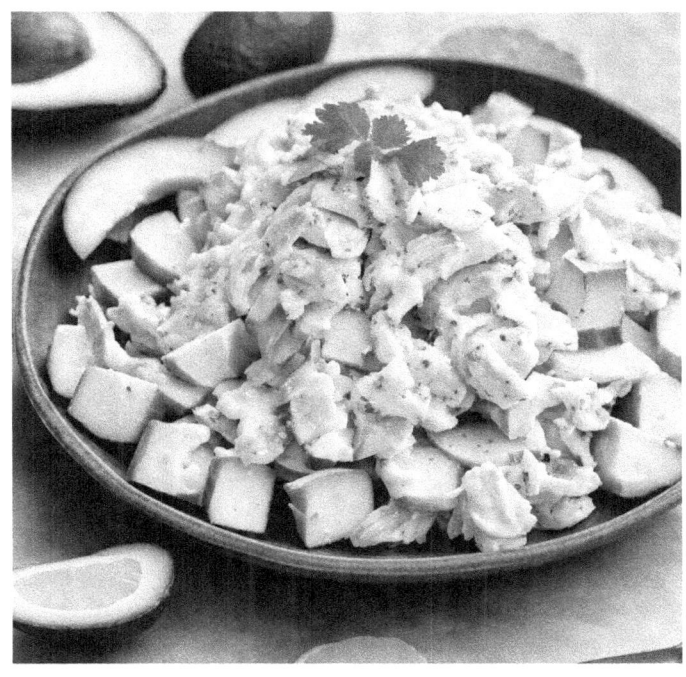

8. Halibut en Papillote

Ingredients:
- 4 halibut fillets (6 ounces each)
- 1 zucchini, thinly sliced
- 1 carrot, thinly sliced
- 1 lemon, thinly sliced
- 4 teaspoons olive oil
- 1/4 cup fresh herbs (parsley, thyme, or basil), chopped

Instructions:
1. Preheat oven to 400°F (200°C).
2. Cut four large squares of parchment paper.
3. On each piece of parchment, place some slices of zucchini, carrot, and a halibut fillet. Top each fillet with lemon slices and 1 teaspoon of olive oil.
4. Sprinkle fresh herbs over the top.
5. Fold parchment paper over the ingredients, crimping edges to seal.
6. Place the packets on a baking sheet and bake for 12-15 minutes, until the fish is cooked through.
7. Carefully open packets (watch for steam) and serve immediately.

Nutrition Info (per serving, serves 4):
- Calories: 220
- Protein: 25 g
- Carbohydrates: 5 g
- Fat: 12 g
- Fiber: 1 g

Cooking Time: 30 minutes

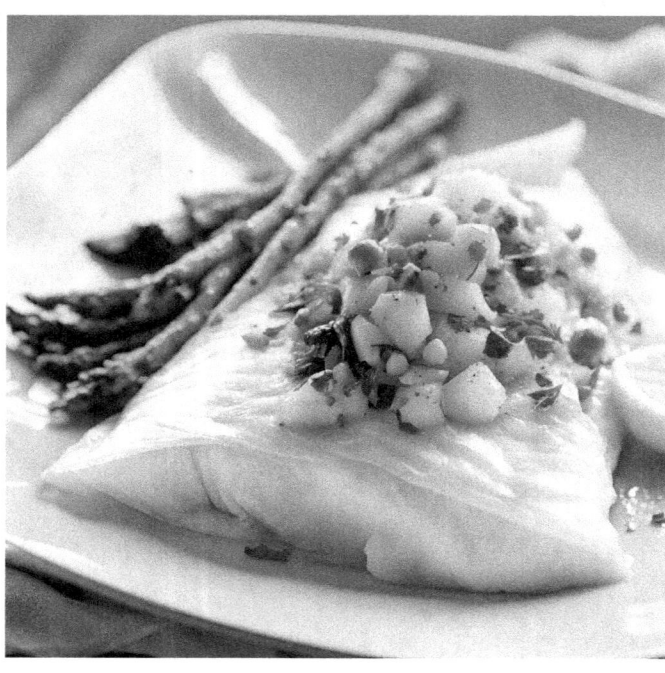

9. Scallops with Cauliflower Puree

Ingredients:
- 1 pound sea scallops
- 1 head cauliflower, cut into florets
- 2 tablespoons olive oil
- 1/2 cup milk (or almond milk)
- 1 garlic clove, minced
- Fresh chives, chopped for garnish

Instructions:
1. Steam cauliflower until very tender, about 10 minutes.
2. In a blender, combine steamed cauliflower, milk, and garlic. Puree until smooth.
3. Heat olive oil in a skillet over medium-high heat. Sear scallops for about 2 minutes on each side until golden and cooked through.
4. Serve scallops over a bed of cauliflower puree and garnish with chives.

Nutrition Info (per serving, serves 4):
- Calories: 220
- Protein: 23 g
- Carbohydrates: 10 g
- Fat: 10 g
- Fiber: 3 g

Cooking Time: 20 minutes

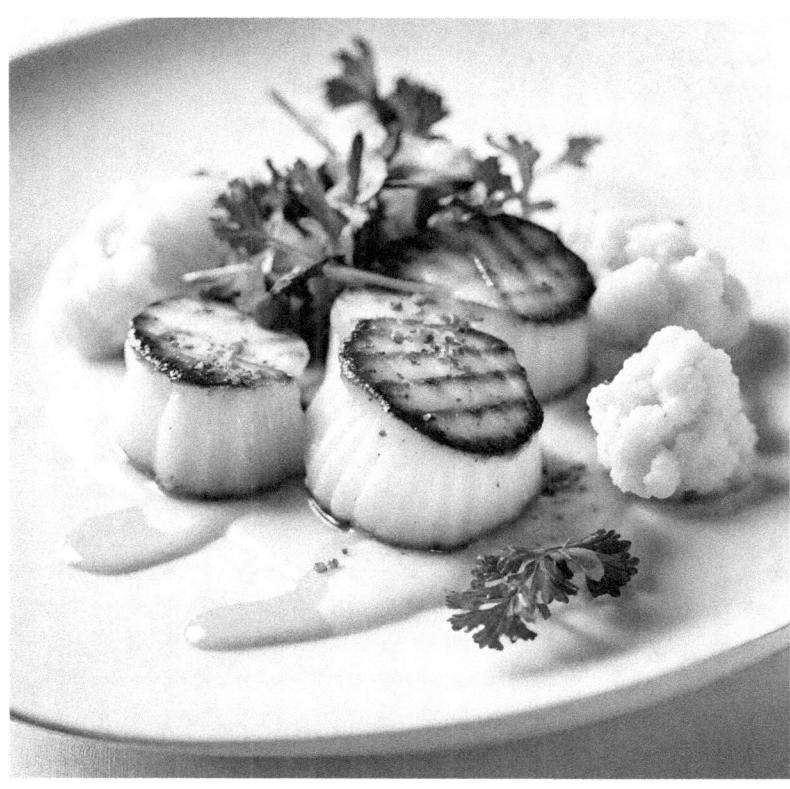

10. Lemon Garlic Tilapia

Ingredients:
- 4 tilapia fillets (6 ounces each)
- 2 lemons, juiced and zest grated
- 3 cloves garlic, minced
- 2 tablespoons olive oil
- Fresh parsley, chopped for garnish

Instructions:
1. Preheat oven to 400°F (200°C).
2. In a small bowl, mix lemon juice, lemon zest, garlic, and olive oil.
3. Place tilapia in a baking dish and pour lemon mixture over the fillets.
4. Bake for 12-15 minutes until fish flakes easily with a fork.
5. Garnish with fresh parsley before serving.

Nutrition Info (per serving, serves 4):
- Calories: 180
- Protein: 23 g
- Carbohydrates: 3 g
- Fat: 9 g
- Fiber: 1 g

Cooking Time: 15 minutes

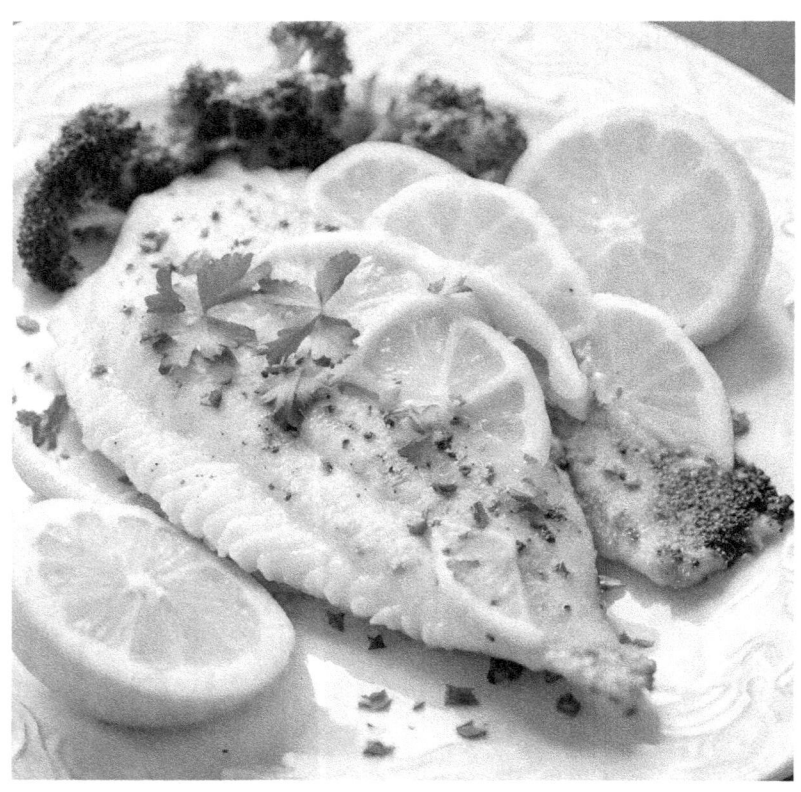

11. Sardine Spread

Ingredients:
- 2 cans sardines in olive oil, drained
- 1/4 cup plain yogurt
- 1 lemon, juiced
- 1 tablespoon capers, chopped
- 1 tablespoon fresh dill, chopped
- Crackers or whole wheat bread for serving

Instructions:
1. In a bowl, mash sardines with a fork.
2. Mix in yogurt, lemon juice, capers, and dill until well combined.
3. Serve on crackers or sliced bread.

Nutrition Info (per serving, serves 4):
- Calories: 180
- Protein: 15 g
- Carbohydrates: 2 g
- Fat: 13 g
- Fiber: 0 g

Cooking Time: 10 minutes

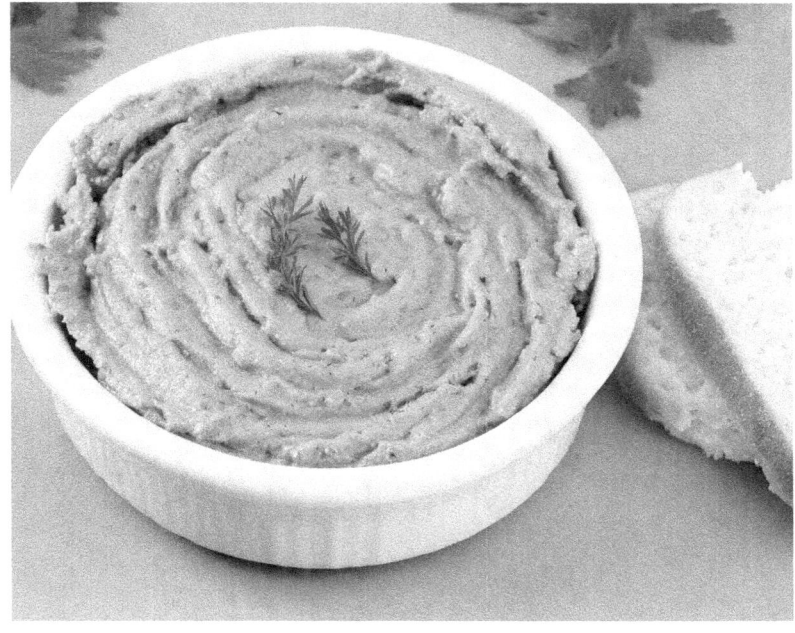

12. Clam Chowder with Sweet Potatoes

Ingredients:
- 2 cups chopped clams, drained
- 2 sweet potatoes, peeled and cubed
- 1 onion, chopped
- 2 celery stalks, chopped
- 4 cups fish or vegetable broth
- 1 cup light cream (or coconut milk)
- 2 tablespoons olive oil
- Fresh thyme, chopped

Instructions:
1. Heat olive oil in a large pot over medium heat. Sauté onion and celery until soft.
2. Add sweet potatoes and broth. Bring to a boil, then simmer until potatoes are tender, about 15 minutes.
3. Add clams and cream. Heat through without boiling.
4. Stir in fresh thyme and serve.

Nutrition Info (per serving, serves 4):
- Calories: 300
- Protein: 18 g
- Carbohydrates: 30 g
- Fat: 14 g
- Fiber: 4 g

Cooking Time: 30 minutes

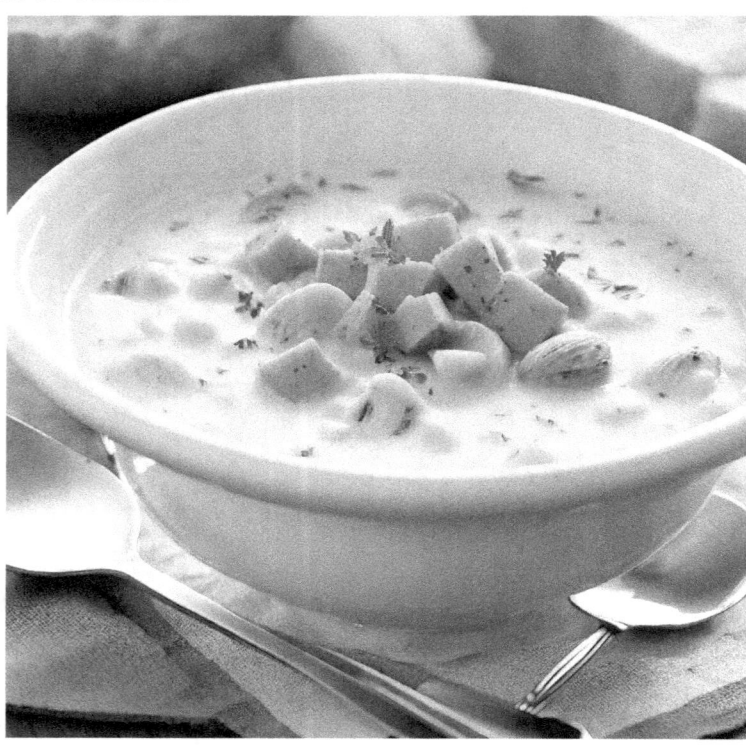

13. Oyster Stew

Ingredients:
- 1 pint fresh oysters, with their liquor
- 2 cups milk
- 1 cup cream
- 1/4 cup butter
- 1 celery stalk, finely chopped
- 1 onion, finely chopped
- 1 tablespoon fresh parsley, chopped
- 1/4 teaspoon paprika

Instructions:
1. In a large saucepan, melt butter over medium heat. Add onion and celery, and sauté until translucent.
2. Add oysters with their liquor. Cook until oysters start to curl at the edges.
3. Pour in milk and cream, gently heat until just below boiling (do not boil).
4. Season with paprika and stir in parsley before serving.

Nutrition Info (per serving, serves 4):
- Calories: 390
- Protein: 16 g
- Carbohydrates: 15 g
- Fat: 30 g
- Fiber: 1 g

Cooking Time: 20 minutes

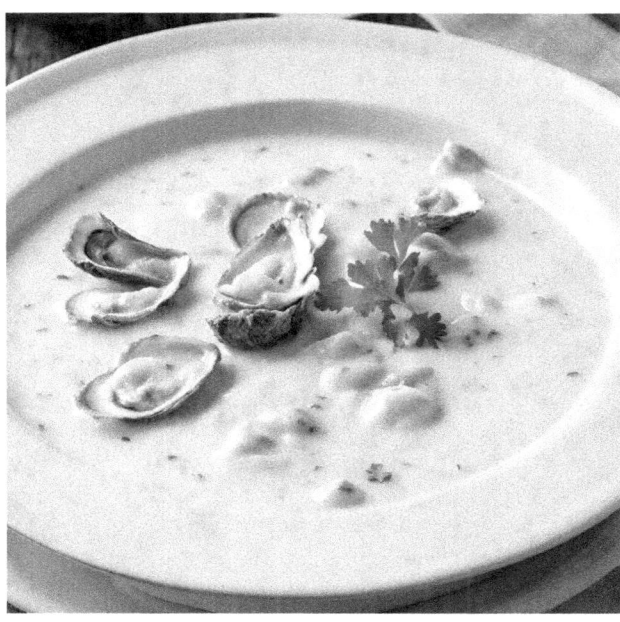

14. Spicy Grilled Octopus

Ingredients:
- 1 octopus, cleaned and tentacles separated
- 2 tablespoons olive oil
- 1 lemon, juiced
- 2 cloves garlic, minced
- 1 teaspoon chili flakes
- Fresh parsley, chopped for garnish

Instructions:
1. Boil octopus in a pot of water for about 20 minutes or until tender. Drain and let cool.
2. In a bowl, mix olive oil, lemon juice, garlic, and chili flakes.
3. Marinate the octopus tentacles in the mixture for at least 30 minutes.
4. Preheat the grill to medium-high heat. Grill octopus for about 4-5 minutes on each side until charred.
5. Garnish with parsley and serve.

Nutrition Info (per serving, serves 4):
- Calories: 200
- Protein: 25 g
- Carbohydrates: 5 g
- Fat: 9 g
- Fiber: 0 g

Cooking Time: 1 hour 10 minutes (including marinating time)

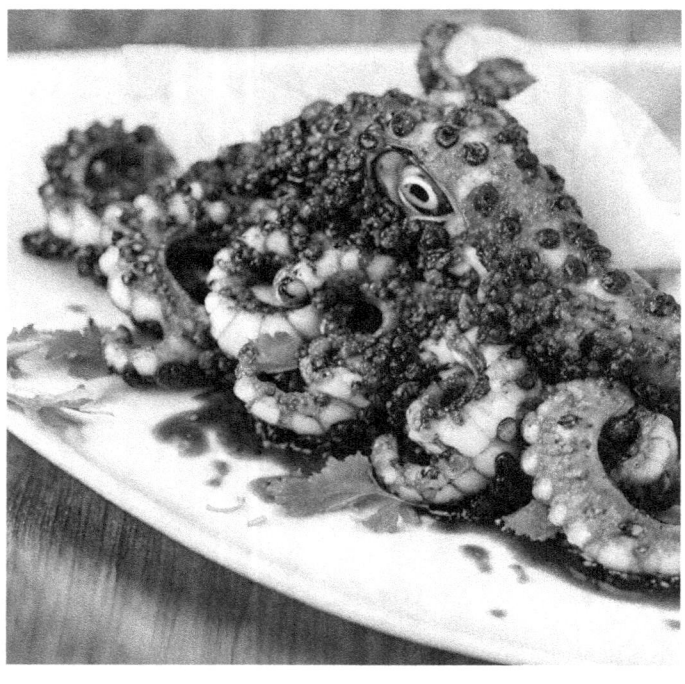

15. Salmon Burgers with Dill Yogurt Sauce

Ingredients:
- 1 pound salmon fillet, skin removed and finely chopped
- 1/2 cup breadcrumbs
- 1 egg
- 2 tablespoons fresh dill, chopped
- 1/2 cup Greek yogurt
- 1 tablespoon lemon juice
- 1 cucumber, grated

Instructions:
1. In a bowl, combine salmon, breadcrumbs, egg, and 1 tablespoon dill. Form into 4 patties.
2. Cook patties in a skillet with a little oil over medium heat, about 4 minutes per side.
3. Mix Greek yogurt, remaining dill, lemon juice, and grated cucumber to make the sauce.
4. Serve salmon burgers with dill yogurt sauce.

Nutrition Info (per serving, serves 4):
- Calories: 290
- Protein: 25 g
- Carbohydrates: 10 g
- Fat: 16 g
- Fiber: 1 g

Cooking Time: 20 minutes

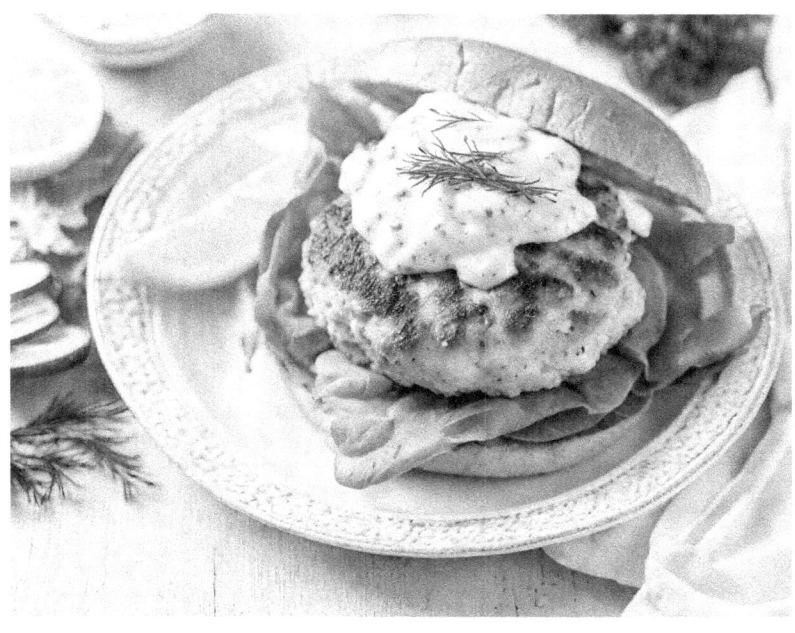

16. Prawn Curry with Coconut Milk

Ingredients:
- 1 pound prawns, peeled and deveined
- 1 can (14 oz) coconut milk
- 1 onion, chopped
- 1 tomato, chopped
- 1 tablespoon curry powder
- 2 cloves garlic, minced
- 2 tablespoons olive oil
- 1/4 cup fresh cilantro, chopped

Instructions:
1. Heat olive oil in a skillet over medium heat. Add onion and garlic, sauté until soft.
2. Stir in curry powder and tomato, cook for 2 minutes.
3. Add prawns and coconut milk, bring to a simmer, and cook until prawns are pink and cooked through, about 5 minutes.
4. Garnish with cilantro and serve.

Nutrition Info (per serving, serves 4):
- Calories: 350
- Protein: 25 g
- Carbohydrates: 8 g
- Fat: 25 g
- Fiber: 2 g

Cooking Time: 20 minutes

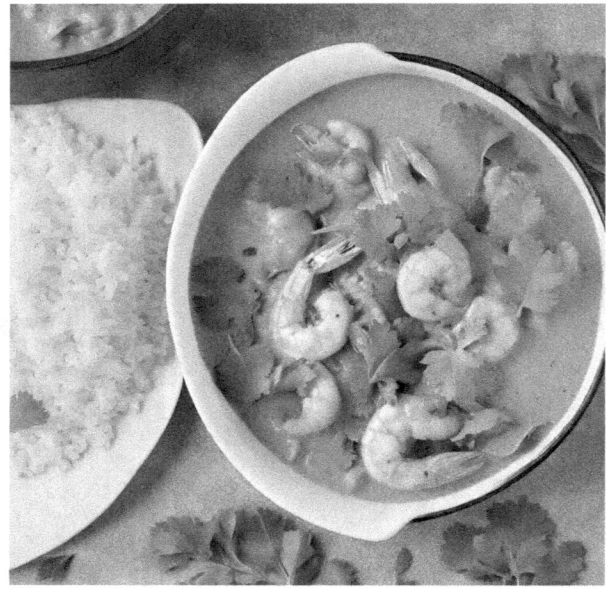

17. Smoked Haddock Omelette

Ingredients:
- 8 ounces smoked haddock, flaked
- 4 eggs
- 1/4 cup milk
- 2 tablespoons butter
- 1 tablespoon fresh chives, chopped
- 1/4 cup grated cheese (optional)

Instructions:
1. In a bowl, whisk together eggs and milk.
2. Melt butter in a non-stick skillet over medium heat.
3. Pour in the egg mixture. As it begins to set, gently pull the edges towards the center, allowing uncooked eggs to flow underneath.
4. When the omelette is almost set, sprinkle flaked haddock and cheese (if using) over half of the omelette.
5. Fold the other half over the filling and slide onto a plate.
6. Garnish with chopped chives and serve.

Nutrition Info (per serving, serves 2):
- Calories: 380
- Protein: 38 g
- Carbohydrates: 2 g
- Fat: 24 g
- Fiber: 0 g

Cooking Time: 15 minutes

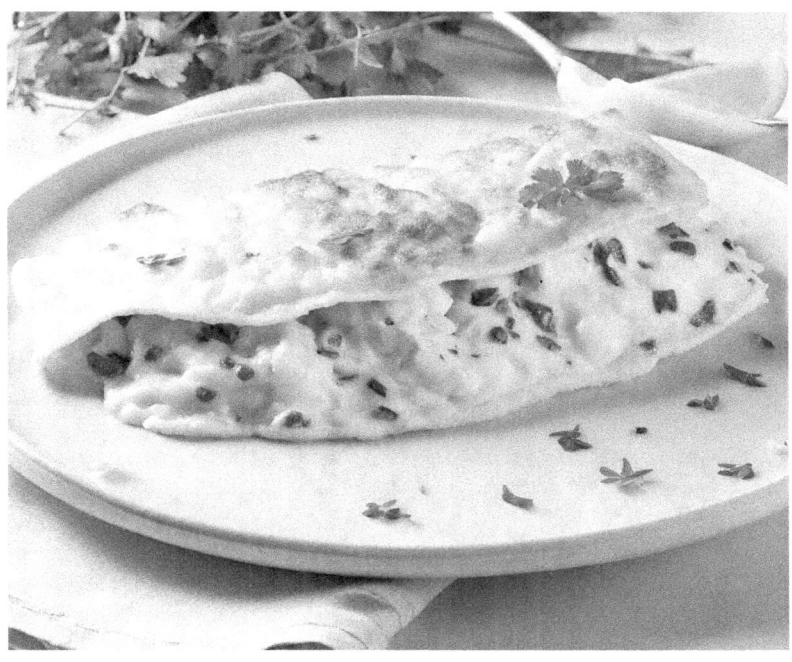

18. Baked Sole with Herb Crust

Ingredients:
- 4 sole fillets (about 6 ounces each)
- 1/2 cup breadcrumbs
- 2 tablespoons olive oil
- 1 lemon, zested and juiced
- 2 tablespoons fresh parsley, chopped
- 1 tablespoon fresh thyme, chopped

Instructions:
1. Preheat oven to 400°F (200°C).
2. In a bowl, mix breadcrumbs, lemon zest, parsley, thyme, and olive oil to form a crumbly mixture.
3. Lay sole fillets on a baking sheet lined with parchment paper.
4. Press the breadcrumb mixture onto each fillet.
5. Bake for 12-15 minutes or until the fish flakes easily with a fork.
6. Drizzle with lemon juice before serving.

Nutrition Info (per serving, serves 4):
- Calories: 230
- Protein: 23 g
- Carbohydrates: 9 g
- Fat: 11 g
- Fiber: 1 g

Cooking Time: 20 minutes

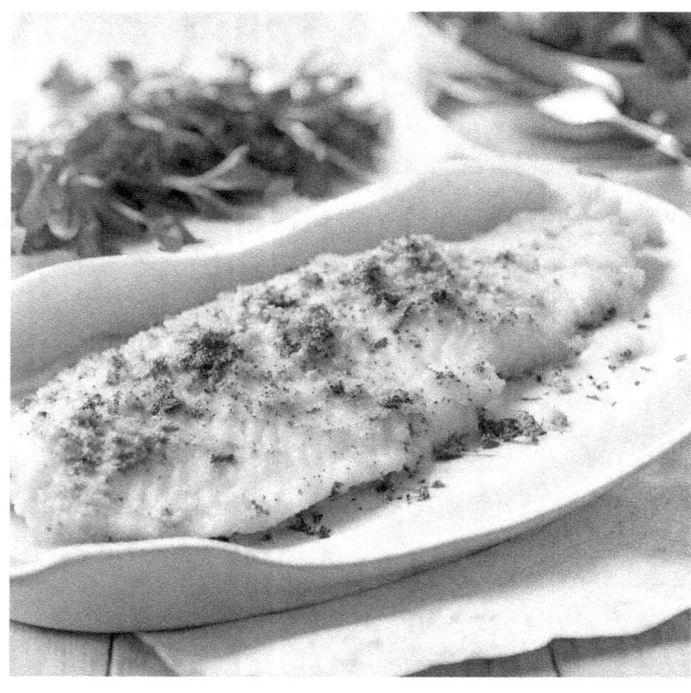

19. Herring in Mustard Sauce

Ingredients:
- 4 herring fillets
- 1/4 cup Dijon mustard
- 1/4 cup white wine vinegar
- 2 tablespoons honey
- 1 tablespoon olive oil
- 1 tablespoon fresh dill, chopped

Instructions:
1. In a small bowl, mix mustard, vinegar, and honey to create the sauce.
2. Lay herring fillets in a shallow dish and pour the sauce over them. Let marinate for at least 30 minutes.
3. Heat olive oil in a skillet over medium heat. Cook herring fillets for about 2-3 minutes on each side or until cooked through.
4. Garnish with fresh dill and serve.

Nutrition Info (per serving, serves 4):
- Calories: 220
- Protein: 20 g
- Carbohydrates: 10 g
- Fat: 10 g
- Fiber: 0 g

Cooking Time: 40 minutes (including marinating time)

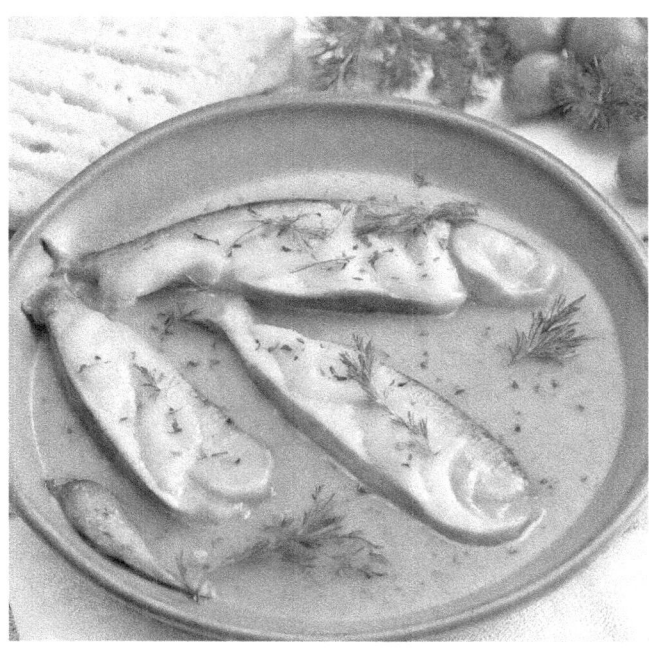

WEEKLY MEAL PLANNER

	BREAKFAST	LUNCH	DINNER	SNACKS
MONDAY				
TUESDAY				
WEDNESDAY				
THURSDAY				
FRIDAY				
SATURDAY				
SUNDAY				

1. What are your current eating habits, and how do you think they affect your Graves' disease symptoms?

WEEKLY MEAL PLANNER

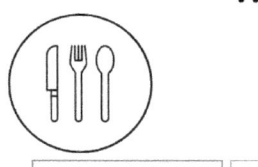

	BREAKFAST	LUNCH	DINNER	SNACKS
MONDAY				
TUESDAY				
WEDNESDAY				
THURSDAY				
FRIDAY				
SATURDAY				
SUNDAY				

Describe a typical day's meals and snacks. Which of these do you think might be impacting your thyroid health positively or negatively?

WEEKLY MEAL PLANNER

	BREAKFAST	LUNCH	DINNER	SNACKS
MONDAY				
TUESDAY				
WEDNESDAY				
THURSDAY				
FRIDAY				
SATURDAY				
SUNDAY				

List any specific foods you currently consume that you know are recommended to avoid with Graves' disease. How do you plan to replace or eliminate these from your diet?

WEEKLY MEAL PLANNER

	BREAKFAST	LUNCH	DINNER	SNACKS
MONDAY				
TUESDAY				
WEDNESDAY				
THURSDAY				
FRIDAY				
SATURDAY				
SUNDAY				

Have you noticed any foods that exacerbate your symptoms? What are they, and how do you plan to manage or avoid them in your diet?

WEEKLY MEAL PLANNER

	BREAKFAST	LUNCH	DINNER	SNACKS
MONDAY				
TUESDAY				
WEDNESDAY				
THURSDAY				
FRIDAY				
SATURDAY				
SUNDAY				

What are your three main goals for starting the Graves' disease diet?

WEEKLY MEAL PLANNER

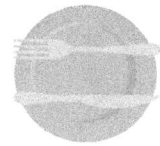

	BREAKFAST	LUNCH	DINNER	SNACKS
MONDAY				
TUESDAY				
WEDNESDAY				
THURSDAY				
FRIDAY				
SATURDAY				
SUNDAY				

Identify three Graves' disease-friendly recipes from the cookbook that you are excited to try. What appeals to you about them?

WEEKLY MEAL PLANNER

	BREAKFAST	LUNCH	DINNER	SNACKS
MONDAY				
TUESDAY				
WEDNESDAY				
THURSDAY				
FRIDAY				
SATURDAY				
SUNDAY				

What challenges do you anticipate in maintaining the Graves' disease diet, and how might you overcome them?

WEEKLY MEAL PLANNER

	BREAKFAST	LUNCH	DINNER	SNACKS
MONDAY				
TUESDAY				
WEDNESDAY				
THURSDAY				
FRIDAY				
SATURDAY				
SUNDAY				

Do you have any concerns about starting this diet? What steps can you take to address these concerns?

WEEKLY MEAL PLANNER

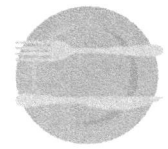

	BREAKFAST	LUNCH	DINNER	SNACKS
MONDAY				
TUESDAY				
WEDNESDAY				
THURSDAY				
FRIDAY				
SATURDAY				
SUNDAY				

After one month on the Graves' disease diet, what improvements or changes in symptoms do you hope to see?

7-WEEK MEAL PLAN

Week 1
Day 1
- **Breakfast:** Quinoa Porridge
- **Lunch:** Chicken Salad
- **Dinner:** Beef Stir-Fry
- **Snack:** Carrot Cake Oatmeal

Day 2
- **Breakfast:** Gluten-Free Oatmeal
- **Lunch:** Beef and Vegetable Soup
- **Dinner:** Grilled Salmon with Lemon and Dill
- **Snack:** Apple Cinnamon Millet Bowl

Day 3
- **Breakfast:** Buckwheat Pancakes
- **Lunch:** Crab Salad with Avocado and Cucumber
- **Dinner:** Pork Tenderloin
- **Snack:** Chia Pudding

Day 4
- **Breakfast:** Smoothie Bowl
- **Lunch:** Italian Meatballs
- **Dinner:** Baked Cod with Olive Tapenade
- **Snack:** Sautéed Greens

Day 5
- **Breakfast:** Chia Pudding
- **Lunch:** Beef Kabobs
- **Dinner:** Pan-Seared Tuna Steaks
- **Snack:** Rice Cakes

Day 6
- **Breakfast:** Baked Sweet Potato
- **Lunch:** Spicy Stir-Fried Cabbage
- **Dinner:** Seafood Paella with Brown Rice
- **Snack:** Almond Flour Crepes

Day 7
- **Breakfast:** Avocado Toast
- **Lunch:** Chicken Vegetable Kebabs
- **Dinner:** Beef Stroganoff
- **Snack:** Pumpkin Porridge

Week 2
Day 8
- **Breakfast:** Egg Muffins
- **Lunch:** Mussels in Tomato Garlic Broth
- **Dinner:** Pork Chops with Apples and Onions
- **Snack:** Greek Yogurt Parfait

Day 9
- **Breakfast:** Turkey Bacon Wraps
- **Lunch:** Stuffed Turkey Breast
- **Dinner:** Chicken Paillard
- **Snack:** Savory Oatmeal

Day 10
- **Breakfast:** Greek Yogurt Parfait
- **Lunch:** Turkey Skillet
- **Dinner:** Chicken Piccata
- **Snack:** Zucchini Bread

Day 11
- **Breakfast:** Savory Oatmeal
- **Lunch:** Roast Chicken with Thyme
- **Dinner:** Turkey Soup
- **Snack:** Almond Flour Crepes

Day 12
- **Breakfast:** Rice Cakes
- **Lunch:** Chicken Caesar Salad
- **Dinner:** Slow Cooker Turkey Breast
- **Snack:** Greek Yogurt Parfait

Day 13
- **Breakfast:** Almond Flour Crepes
- **Lunch:** Turkey and Vegetable Stew
- **Dinner:** Grilled Chicken Caesar Wrap
- **Snack:** Pumpkin Porridge

Day 14
- **Breakfast:** Pumpkin Porridge
- **Lunch:** Lemon Garlic Turkey Cutlets
- **Dinner:** Grilled Chicken Salad
- **Snack:** Zucchini Bread

Week 3

Day 15
- **Breakfast:** Zucchini Bread
- **Lunch:** Turkey Meatballs
- **Dinner:** Shrimp Stir-Fry with Mixed Vegetables
- **Snack:** Savory Oatmeal

Day 16
- **Breakfast:** Savory Oatmeal
- **Lunch:** Chicken Stir-Fry
- **Dinner:** Roasted Turkey Breast
- **Snack:** Almond Flour Crepes

Day 17
- **Breakfast:** Rice Cakes
- **Lunch:** Pork and Sweet Potato Stew
- **Dinner:** Balsamic Glazed Beef
- **Snack:** Greek Yogurt Parfait

Day 18
- **Breakfast:** Almond Flour Crepes
- **Lunch:** Spiced Pork Ribs
- **Dinner:** Beef Bourguignon
- **Snack:** Pumpkin Porridge

Day 19
- **Breakfast:** Pumpkin Porridge
- **Lunch:** Pork Scallopini
- **Dinner:** Beef Chili
- **Snack:** Zucchini Bread

Day 20
- **Breakfast:** Zucchini Bread
- **Lunch:** Ginger Pork Stir-Fry
- **Dinner:** Beef Brisket
- **Snack:** Savory Oatmeal

Day 21
- **Breakfast:** Savory Oatmeal
- **Lunch:** Pork Carnitas
- **Dinner:** Beef Tenderloin with Herb Crust
- **Snack:** Almond Flour Crepes

Week 4
Day 22
- **Breakfast:** Baked Sole with Herb Crust
- **Lunch:** Chicken Vegetable Soup
- **Dinner:** Pork Vegetable Soup
- **Snack:** Apple Cinnamon Millet Bowl

Day 23
- **Breakfast:** Greek Yogurt Parfait
- **Lunch:** Beef Goulash
- **Dinner:** Salmon Burgers with Dill Yogurt Sauce
- **Snack:** Chia Pudding

Day 24
- **Breakfast:** Smoothie Bowl
- **Lunch:** Spicy Grilled Octopus
- **Dinner:** Prawn Curry with Coconut Milk
- **Snack:** Rice Cakes

Day 25
- **Breakfast:** Egg Muffins
- **Lunch:** Smoked Haddock Omelette
- **Dinner:** Sardine Spread
- **Snack:** Greek Yogurt Parfait

Day 26
- **Breakfast:** Gluten-Free Oatmeal
- **Lunch:** Sea Bass with Fennel and Orange
- **Dinner:** Clam Chowder with Sweet Potatoes
- **Snack:** Almond Flour Crepes

Day 27
- **Breakfast:** Buckwheat Pancakes
- **Lunch:** Herring in Mustard Sauce
- **Dinner:** Oyster Stew
- **Snack:** Pumpkin Porridge

Day 28
- **Breakfast:** Avocado Toast
- **Lunch:** Halibut en Papillote
- **Dinner:** Scallop with Cauliflower Puree
- **Snack:** Zucchini Bread

Week 5

Day 29
- **Breakfast:** Quinoa Porridge
- **Lunch:** Lemon Garlic Tilapia
- **Dinner:** Grilled Salmon with Lemon and Dill
- **Snack:** Carrot Cake Oatmeal

Day 30
- **Breakfast:** Baked Sweet Potato
- **Lunch:** Beef Stroganoff
- **Dinner:** Pork Tenderloin
- **Snack:** Apple Cinnamon Millet Bowl

Day 31
- **Breakfast:** Avocado Toast
- **Lunch:** Turkey Skillet
- **Dinner:** Chicken Caesar Salad
- **Snack:** Greek Yogurt Parfait

Day 32
- **Breakfast:** Gluten-Free Oatmeal
- **Lunch:** Turkey Meatballs
- **Dinner:** Beef and Vegetable Soup
- **Snack:** Savory Oatmeal

Day 33
- **Breakfast:** Buckwheat Pancakes
- **Lunch:** Chicken Stir-Fry
- **Dinner:** Spicy Stir-Fried Cabbage
- **Snack:** Zucchini Bread

Day 34
- **Breakfast:** Smoothie Bowl
- **Lunch:** Roast Chicken with Thyme
- **Dinner:** Slow Cooker Turkey Breast
- **Snack:** Almond Flour Crepes

Day 35
- **Breakfast:** Egg Muffins
- **Lunch:** Turkey and Vegetable Stew
- **Dinner:** Grilled Chicken Caesar Wrap
- **Snack:** Pumpkin Porridge

Week 6

Day 36
- **Breakfast:** Greek Yogurt Parfait
- **Lunch:** Lemon Garlic Turkey Cutlets
- **Dinner:** Beef Chili
- **Snack:** Chia Pudding

Day 37
- **Breakfast:** Savory Oatmeal
- **Lunch:** Pork Carnitas
- **Dinner:** Beef Tenderloin with Herb Crust
- **Snack:** Rice Cakes

Day 38
- **Breakfast:** Rice Cakes
- **Lunch:** Ginger Pork Stir-Fry
- **Dinner:** Beef Brisket
- **Snack:** Greek Yogurt Parfait

Day 39
- **Breakfast:** Almond Flour Crepes
- **Lunch:** Grilled Chicken Salad
- **Dinner:** Turkey Soup
- **Snack:** Pumpkin Porridge

Day 40
- **Breakfast:** Pumpkin Porridge
- **Lunch:** Spicy Grilled Octopus
- **Dinner:** Prawn Curry with Coconut Milk
- **Snack:** Zucchini Bread

Day 41
- **Breakfast:** Zucchini Bread
- **Lunch:** Smoked Haddock Omelette
- **Dinner:** Salmon Burgers with Dill Yogurt Sauce
- **Snack:** Savory Oatmeal

Day 42
- **Breakfast:** Savory Oatmeal
- **Lunch:** Herring in Mustard Sauce
- **Dinner:** Sea Bass with Fennel and Orange
- **Snack:** Almond Flour Crepes

Week 7

Day 43
- **Breakfast:** Gluten-Free Oatmeal
- **Lunch:** Beef Stroganoff
- **Dinner:** Grilled Salmon with Lemon and Dill
- **Snack:** Carrot Cake Oatmeal

Day 44
- **Breakfast:** Buckwheat Pancakes
- **Lunch:** Chicken Caesar Salad
- **Dinner:** Pork Tenderloin
- **Snack:** Apple Cinnamon Millet Bowl

Day 45
- **Breakfast:** Smoothie Bowl
- **Lunch:** Turkey Meatballs
- **Dinner:** Beef and Vegetable Soup
- **Snack:** Greek Yogurt Parfait

Day 46
- **Breakfast:** Avocado Toast
- **Lunch:** Roast Chicken with Thyme
- **Dinner:** Slow Cooker Turkey Breast
- **Snack:** Savory Oatmeal

Day 47
- **Breakfast:** Egg Muffins
- **Lunch:** Turkey and Vegetable Stew
- **Dinner:** Grilled Chicken Caesar Wrap
- **Snack:** Zucchini Bread

Day 48
- **Breakfast:** Baked Sweet Potato
- **Lunch:** Spicy Stir-Fried Cabbage
- **Dinner:** Beef Chili
- **Snack:** Almond Flour Crepes

Day 49
- **Breakfast:** Greek Yogurt Parfait
- **Lunch:** Lemon Garlic Turkey Cutlets
- **Dinner:** Pork Carnitas
- **Snack:** Chia Pudding

SCAN THE QR CODE BELOW TO GET YOUR E-BOOK WITH FULL COLOR PICTURES

www.ingramcontent.com/pod-product-compliance
Lightning Source LLC
Chambersburg PA
CBHW082206220526
45470CB00010B/3058